EMPATHIC ENGAGEMENT IN CLINICAL PRACTICE

Here is a book on empathy that is simultaneously theoretically sophisticated and highly practical. This refreshing new look at empathy describes how imaginative entry into the world of the other leads to the erasing of self–other boundaries and immersion in the client's inner world. Empathic engagement with the client from this inside vantage point leads to a reduction in the client's feeling of the therapist as an outsider and facilitates the client feeling safe and open. This book provides both theoretical explication of and practical skills for how to participate in this type of empathic engagement. It is a must-read for anyone interested in the process, the power, and the use of empathy in therapy, and is a highly worthwhile read for practitioners of all persuasions.

—**Leslie S. Greenberg, PhD,** Distinguished Research Professor Emeritus, Department of Psychology, York University, Toronto, ON, Canada

Since Carl Rogers's early advocacy of empathy as key to effective therapy, confusion has followed about its meaning and professional use. Flemons clears up this confusion, drawing on useful everyday resources as well as providing recommendations derived from clinical research to enhance professional relationships, in ways that also promote better professional self-care.

—**Tom Strong, MEd, PhD,** psychologist and professor emeritus, Counselling Psychology, University of Calgary, Calgary, AB, Canada

Douglas Flemons has taken on the seemingly impossible task of defining the nature of empathy, identifying its core components, and teaching the skills that are foundational to good psychotherapy. He has succeeded in every way! This is a book that considers empathy from many different current and historical perspectives, challenges conventional wisdom, and pokes at standard techniques that may sound reasonable but don't work all that well in real-life scenarios. The inspiring and practical perspectives and methods Flemons offers in this carefully crafted book deserve the attention of anyone and everyone who grasps the value of a meaningful connection with another human being.

—**Michael D. Yapko, PhD,** clinical psychologist and author of *Trancework* (6th ed.) and *The Discriminating Therapist*

This book is a prism. It will not only help you to understand others but to help them feel understood by you.

—**Daryl Chow, PhD,** author of *Crossing Between Worlds* and writer on Substack, *Full Circles: Field Notes on the Inner and Outer Life*

Clearly written and carefully researched, this book will make you rethink what empathy is and how therapists and other health professionals can use it to promote therapeutic ends. A masterful weaving of current psychological research, philosophy of mind and neuroscience, and insights from decades of clinical experience, makes this short and accessible book a must-read for health professionals aspiring to be more effective and relationally attuned with their patients and clients. Highly recommended.

—**Ronald Epstein, MD,** University of Rochester, Rochester, NY, United States; author of *Attending: Medicine, Mindfulness, and Humanity*

EMPATHIC ENGAGEMENT IN CLINICAL PRACTICE

DOUGLAS FLEMONS

 AMERICAN PSYCHOLOGICAL ASSOCIATION

Copyright © 2026 by the American Psychological Association. All rights, including for text and data mining, AI training, and similar technologies, are reserved. Except as permitted under the United States Copyright Act of 1976, no part of this publication may be reproduced or distributed in any form or by any means, including, but not limited to, the process of scanning and digitization, or stored in a database or retrieval system, without the prior written permission of the publisher.

The opinions and statements published are those of the Author, and do not necessarily represent the policies of the American Psychological Association. The information contained in this work does not constitute personalized therapeutic advice. Users seeking medical advice, diagnoses, or treatment should consult a medical professional or health care provider. The Author has worked to ensure that all information in this book is accurate at the time of publication and consistent with general mental health care standards.

Published by
American Psychological Association
750 First Street, NE
Washington, DC 20002
https://www.apa.org

Order Department
https://www.apa.org/pubs/books
order@apa.org

Typeset in Charter and Interstate by Circle Graphics, Inc., Reisterstown, MD

Printer: Vicks Lithograph & Printing, Yorkville, NY
Cover Designer: Gwen J. Grafft, Minneapolis, MN

Library of Congress Cataloging-in-Publication Data

Names: Flemons, Douglas G. author
Title: Empathic engagement in clinical practice / by Douglas Flemons.
Description: Washington, D.C. : American Psychological Association, [2026] | Includes bibliographical references and index.
Identifiers: LCCN 2025018119 (print) | LCCN 2025018120 (ebook) | ISBN 9781433843365 paperback | ISBN 9781433843372 ebook
Subjects: LCSH: Psychotherapist and patient | Empathy | BISAC: PSYCHOLOGY / Clinical Psychology
Classification: LCC RC480.8 .F58 2026 (print) | LCC RC480.8 (ebook)
LC record available at https://lccn.loc.gov/2025018119
LC ebook record available at https://lccn.loc.gov/2025018120

ISBN 9781433849961 (pdf)

https://doi.org/10.1037/0000472-000

Printed in the United States of America

10 9 8 7 6 5 4 3 2 1

To Shelley, with whom life makes sense.

*We live storied lives. . . . Our identities—who we are and what we do—
originate in the tales passed down to us and the stories we take on as our
own. In this sense, stories constitute "our medium of being." . . . Storytelling
is both a method of knowing . . . and a way of telling about our lives.*
—Arthur P. Bochner, Coming to Narrative (2014, p. 293)

*Perhaps the triumphal assumption that we can easily understand one another
is as sinful as the refusal to attempt any human understanding at all, and
that would mean that our obligation is to try grasping one another in the
full realization that it cannot be done with complete success.*
—Ted Cohen, Thinking of Others: On the Talent for Metaphor (2008, p. 70)

*Empathy has been credited with the power to shift the shape of the self so
as to enter into alien forms, to transform into art objects, to inhabit other
realities, and to take on the experiences of other persons. To look back at
empathy in all its varieties is to witness, directly and obliquely, the diffusion
of the self across its feeling connections.*
—Susan Lanzoni, Empathy: A History (2018, p. 2)

Contents

Acknowledgments	*xi*
Introduction: The Process of Empathy	3
1. The Invention, Evolution, and Differentiation of Empathy	11
2. Developing Empathic Curiosity	41
3. Practicing Therapist Self-Care	73
4. Orienting Empathically to Clients	93
5. Skills of Empathic Engagement	119
Epilogue: Circling Back and Heading Out	*159*
References	*165*
Index	*189*
About the Author	*195*

Acknowledgments

I'm grateful for the community of family, friends, colleagues, students, teachers, and clients whose contributions to my life and understanding made this book possible.

My keen-eyed wife, Shelley Green, was my first and final reader, helping me recognize what did and didn't yet make sense. My brother, Ward, and son, Eric, each closely read and talked with me at length about the fine details. A small cadre of friends—Steve Alford, Ray Becvar, Greg Blom, Monte Bobele, Art Bochner, Brit Davis, Carolyn Ellis, Suzanne Ferriss, Eric Greenleaf, Mog Hesthammer, Martha Laughlin, Scott Miller, Michael Reiter, Sandra Roscoe, Tom Strong, and Michael Yapko—generously provided detailed feedback and encouragement at various stages along the way. Other colleagues and friends, including Jason DeCristafaro, Lori Finley, Jerry Gale, James and Valerie Judd, Adam Saslov, and Kathee and David Todtman, offered personal anecdotes and invaluable nuggets of professional wisdom. Jenna Flemons put the ideas into practice in her new career as a therapist. Ken Wood gave me permission to write about his demonstration of unflappable empathy in a trying circumstance. Carolyn Ellis told me the moving personal story that begins Chapter 1. She kindly gave me permission to recount it, and she and her husband, Art Bochner, ensured that my rendering accurately captured their experience.

I was introduced to the concept and practice of empathy during my master's Counselling Psychology Program at the University of British Columbia. Several faculty members, including John Banmen, Bill Borgen, Larry Cochrane,

Les Greenberg, Dianne Pollard, and Marv Westwood, helped me develop my nascent clinical understanding and professional commitment to compassionate care.

I was first inspired to bring empathy into foreground focus by two of my doctoral students, Victoria Lazarev and Brit Davis. Subsequent in-depth conversations with Brit and her brother Greg fired me up to write an article for the *Psychotherapy Networker*, which subsequently expanded and morphed into a book prospectus, which, thanks to Scott Miller, I was fortunate enough to send to Susan Reynolds at the American Psychological Association. Susan helped me shape my proposal into a workable plan, and David Becker helped me distill the submitted manuscript into a coherent whole. Each of them was assisted by discerning anonymous reviewers, who devoted considerable time and focused attention to improving the text. Erin O'Brien caught my mistakes and fine-tuned my sentences.

The novelist E. M. Forster once told a story about an old lady who exclaimed to her nieces, "How can I tell what I think till I see what I say?" I'm with her: Writing is such a rich source of discovery. But then, so is speaking—I often don't have a good grasp of what I think or know until I hear myself saying it. For this reason, I have welcomed offers over the last few years to give talks or workshops on empathy in a variety of settings. I'm grateful for opportunities extended by Victoria Lazarev, Ward Flemons and Jane Lemaire, Jeff Krepps and Cheyenne Corbett, Judith Leemann and Kenneth Bailey, and, most recently, Martha Laughlin and Kate Warner.

Finally, I thank the devoted and resourceful librarians who staff Nova Southeastern University's excellent electronic library. They expeditiously tracked down and sent me everything I needed.

EMPATHIC ENGAGEMENT IN CLINICAL PRACTICE

INTRODUCTION
The Process of Empathy

> *If we locate empathy "in" the therapist, in only one part of the therapeutic system, we are ignoring the process, the patterns of interaction between therapist and client(s).*
> —Mary Wilkinson, *How Do We Understand Empathy Systemically?* (1992, p. 194)

This book provides the means for you to think and feel your way into a body–mind appreciation of what empathy is and how it works, an understanding to bring with you into your clinical practice, into what you do and say in conversation with your clients or patients.[1] Whether you're a psychotherapist or a health care professional, learning how to empathize effectively can be a game changer, improving your relationship with those you're trying to help and enhancing your capacity to make a difference.

---

[1] I don't like either word. As I've said elsewhere (Flemons & Gralnik, 2013), *client* is burdened by problematic business-forward overtones, and *patient* fails to evoke the agency and resourcefulness of the people who reach out to us for assistance. With no nonannoying alternative available, I mostly use *client* throughout the book, save for when I refer more specifically to help seekers in a medical context.

https://doi.org/10.1037/0000472-001
Empathic Engagement in Clinical Practice, by D. Flemons
Copyright © 2026 by the American Psychological Association. All rights reserved.

Although I wrote this book for clinicians, empathy is not our exclusive domain. Poets, actors, novelists, historians, philosophers (both Western and Eastern), brain researchers, and meditation teachers also have much to contribute to understanding how to understand another person empathically. Approaching the book as an interdisciplinary dialogue, I've woven quotes throughout the text from a wide range of relevant experts.

Empathy is a way of coming to understand the sense and sensibility of clients, not from some supposed "objective" (outside) vantage but, rather, from inside the logic of their intra- and interpersonal relationships. Developing an insider's grasp of a client's world involves firing up your curiosity and projecting your imagination into the heart of the person's experience, as well as empathically engaging them in conversation. You ask questions and listen closely to the client's answers; you give voice to how you're making sense of what they tell you; and then, responsive to their feedback, you adapt and refine your understanding accordingly. It is a profoundly interactive, intimate process of discovering, inferring, and sharing, one that demands compassionate presence, active listening, and immersive focus. With this in mind, I've done my best to create a reading experience for you that is in some ways isomorphic to this casually conversational yet precision-tuned nature of empathy, one that evokes its friendly informality and storytelling, while closely attending to nuances of meaning in what people say and how they say it. I hope what you read intrigues you and stimulates your curiosity; however (and consider this a rigor warning), I expect it may occasionally also fry your brain and belie your assumptions.

As I describe in Chapter 1, the idea of empathy has, from the get-go, been confounding those who research and write about it. As early as 1935, the psychoanalyst Theodor Reik was already griping that "the concept of empathy in psychological discussion has come to mean so much that it is beginning to mean nothing" (as cited in Pigman, 1995, p. 237). Ninety years later, conceptual and terminological disputes and confusions continue to swirl. Part of the problem can be traced to ambiguities embedded within the word itself, so that "to speak of empathy has on occasion been as senseless as to discuss sitting in a box without distinguishing whether one means a compartment in a theater, the driver's seat, or a big case" (Reik, 1948, p. 350). Empathy involves deriving a first-person, embodied understanding of another person's context and experience—their circumstances, their relationship with self and others, and their ways of orienting to both. In the first chapter, I set out to derive an analogous understanding of the word *empathy* itself—its history, its differences from and relationship to related terms (sympathy, compassion, and others), and its relevance to the therapeutic process.

As a therapist, I've always been committed to recommissioning and repurposing items of experience—symptoms—that clients initially assume they'd be better off without (e.g., Flemons, 2002, 2022). I brought this sensibility into researching and writing this book, looking at empathy with an eye to refurbishing it. I was inspired in this venture by a metaphorically intriguing nugget of advice offered in passing by the philosopher Ludwig Wittgenstein (1980): "Sometimes an expression has to be withdrawn from language and sent for cleaning," he said, and "then it can be put back into circulation" (p. 39e). The Zen teacher Shunryu Suzuki (2006) offered similar guidance to those wishing to study Buddhism. He said such an undertaking should involve "a general house cleaning of your mind. You should take everything out of your room and clean it thoroughly" (Suzuki, 2006, p. 111).

You could read the following pages as an elaborated response to Wittgenstein and Suzuki's suggestions; however, as you'll see, I've kept empathy in circulation throughout, and rather than sending it *out* for *cleaning*, I've aimed for an *in-house reconfiguring*. In Chapter 1, I straddle the weird divide between word and concept—between the term empathy and the concept it conveys. Keeping my eye on both, I approach the crisis of meaning in the field by questioning and offering alternatives to some fundamental assumptions widely and often unquestioningly held by researchers and theorists, assumptions about the nature of mind, language, emotion, communication, and the boundaries and constitution of the self. Wittgenstein (1980) endorsed this method of addressing and resolving intractable confusions: "Getting hold on the difficulty *deep down* is what is hard," he said,

> because if it is grasped near the surface it simply remains the difficulty it was. It has to be pulled out by the roots; and that involves our beginning to think about these things in a new way. . . .
>
> Once the new way of thinking has been established, the old problems vanish; indeed they become hard to recapture. For they go with our way of expressing ourselves and, if we clothe ourselves in a new form of expression, the old problems are discarded along with the old garment. (p. 48e)

In my reconfiguring, I've been guided by two quotes that, on the surface, contradict each other, one by the Zen teacher Bernie Glassman and the other by the anthropologist and ecosystemic philosopher Gregory Bateson. Glassman once made a pitch for keeping explanations simple and direct:

> My Ph.D. is in applied mathematics. My advisor used to say, "If you can't explain it, you don't know it." If you can't put it in regular, simple language that people can understand, then you don't really know what you're talking about. (Bridges & Glassman, 2012, pp. 105–106)

I agree; however, sometimes commonly accepted terms and conceptions obscure rather than communicate clarity. Bateson cautioned that "the conventional language in which people talk about [human relations] . . . is mainly a blinding and misleading language, that the metaphors used are in general inappropriate" (as cited in Kirschenbaum & Henderson, 1989a, p. 193). Holding Glassman and Bateson's injunctions in dynamic juxtaposition, I have aimed to make the book accessible, and I have chosen my words carefully, recognizing that the tacit assumptions baked into our thinking and speaking as usual—including the underlying and unrecognized conceptual metaphors that pervade our language (Lakoff & Johnson, 1980)—can trip us up and take us down. I hope that any unconventional terms or phrases or unorthodox renderings of ideas will remind you, the reader, to embrace uncertainty and question your assumptions, both of which are critical not only to understanding empathy but also to employing it in clinical practice.

We think, experience the world, and come to know ourselves and others empathically through stories. I use them throughout the book as idea-delivery systems. Again and again, they help me depict abstract notions and important concepts in a form that is relatable, digestible, and memorable. Right off the top, I introduce you to the emotional whiplash my friend Carolyn Ellis endured in the living room of a bereaved friend; I offer some miniscenarios to tease out the shape-shifting nature of the self; and to help you get a feel for the line that divides self and other—the boundary that empathy, sympathy, and compassion each help you cross—I describe an experiment with soup that I once undertook in a restaurant. From there, I invite you to conduct an experiment of your own involving mindfulness meditation; I ask you to imagine singing in a choir, and then I tell you about the time I tried, and failed, to hoodwink my sister-in-law back in the 1980s. See what I mean? The unfolding discussion is more exploratory conversation than equation, the shape of it more resembling the gathering and sharing of information in a therapy session than the listing of bullet points in a slide presentation.

Taken together, the stories and experiments are invitations for you to derive not just a conceptual appreciation but also an experiential grasp of what empathy is and how it works—to make sense of it and get it in your bones. This is in keeping with what empathy invites and allows—positioning your imagination to facilitate making sense of the client's mind and embodied experience.

Without imagination, there would be no empathy. Chapter 2 explores how you, curious about the client's world, can best imagine your way into it. Authors have long worried about threats to the self that result from the imaginative efforts to understand another empathically. I offer a way of thinking about and undertaking empathic engagement that protects your well-being and your relationship with the client.

I don't remember any of my graduate school professors talking to me or my fellow students about the personal challenges we would face as a result of our empathically connecting with suffering people. This was a long time ago, before there was much cultural recognition of the risks of professional burnout. Chapter 3 offers the self-care guidance I could have used when I first entered the field. Many years into my career, I became the director of a university student counseling center, supervising a dedicated staff working with an onslaught of often highly distressed clients. In addition to our daytime responsibilities, we staffed a 24/7 crisis line for the university. The therapists took calls for a week at a time; their supervisors and I were never without our dedicated cell phones, which could and did ring at any time. We supported and helped a lot of people, but the emotional demands of doing so were, at times, considerable. It was that experience that alerted me to the necessity of proactively protecting the well-being of therapeutic first responders. I wish my wake-up call had happened sooner because I could have then shared the ideas and practices from this chapter with my staff on their first day of employment.

As therapists, we've all seen clients caught in tragic loops, expending great efforts to solve a problem that only exacerbates it. As a supervisor, I've witnessed therapists caught in analogous tragic loops with their clients, in which their heartfelt efforts to empathically connect end up alienating the person they're trying to reach. In Chapter 4, I detail five orienting commitments for empathic engagement that can help you avoid such ironic tangles: distinguishing professional from personal intimacy, accepting the limits of knowing, not presuming that you know, remaining nonjudgmental, and committing to demonstrating, rather than claiming, empathic understanding.

As you read, you'll see that I approach empathy not as an individual trait or a state of being but, rather, as a particular kind of relationship between self and other and as a means of engagement between a therapist and client. Empathy is something you do. Chapter 5 is devoted to helping you develop your empathic skills, not only when working with individuals but also with couples, families, and groups. I demonstrate how to listen empathically, adapting and refining your understanding in response to client feedback; how to ask questions and float hunches; how to effectively intersperse your empathic contributions throughout conversations; how to practice what I call "both–and empathizing" (holding and articulating two or more divergent views or perspectives simultaneously); and how you can weave your therapeutic sensibility into your empathic offerings, finding ways to explicitly acknowledge what the client is experiencing while implicitly establishing resources and potentiating possibilities for change.

One more comment about that rigor warning: In the first two chapters, I methodically build the theoretical and research scaffolding for the practice-based guidance of the last three. If you prefer to know why before you venture into what and how, a deep dive into the first third of the book will satisfy that curiosity. However, if you want to cut to the chase and don't need a rationale for trying something new, then rather than closely following the explorations and explanations of Chapters 1 and 2, you may find a more cursory read suffices. You can always go back to them later if need be.

We're just about ready for blast off, but first, I want to tell you about an interaction between a skilled and experienced colleague of mine, Sebastian, and a client, Nathan, who he had dubbed, in the privacy of his mind, "The Bully."[2] Nathan was a big, brash professor at one of the universities in Boston and the author of half a dozen important books on politics and history. Nathan intimidated his students and colleagues, poked fun at anyone who didn't "measure up," and became loud and threatening when fighting with his wife. When a previous therapist, someone whom Nathan liked, had told him that such abusive behavior was unacceptable, Nathan fired him on the spot. Only one person, an older friend and colleague, had ever been able to "call him on his shit," but after he died, Nathan deemed no one a peer.

In one of their weekly sessions, Nathan lamented to Sebastian about his oldest son leaving for college. Rather than staying in the northeast, the son had decided to go to Stanford, and Nathan was steamed. "Why move all the way across the country," he had angrily demanded of his son, "when you can get twice the education down the street!?"

To enhance their therapeutic alliance, to help Nathan make sense of his inner turmoil, and to perhaps shift him away from lashing out at his son, Sebastian was inspired to share an empathic understanding of Nathan's plight. Having long admired the work of Irvin Yalom (2002), a psychiatrist who advocates therapist transparency and self-disclosure, Sebastian delivered this understanding by way of a personal anecdote.

"So listen," he said warmly, "I know something about what you're going through. I struggled, too, when our oldest daughter decided to go to college out of state. It felt personal, somehow, like she was wanting to get as far away from us as possible. I was surprised by how hurt and angry I felt, but

---

[2]This and all the other case examples throughout the book have been modified to protect the confidentiality and disguise the identities of the individuals described.

I came to realize that I was afraid of losing her to her adulthood, afraid of missing her, and afraid that my wife and I were about to become bit players in her life."

Nathan took a breath, looked up at the ceiling to his left, paused, looked up to the ceiling to his right, and then fixed Sebastian with a stare that bore through his skull. "So tell me," he said, "am I paying *you* for this session, or are you paying *me*?" Sebastian, feeling about two inches tall, explained that he was merely trying to show him that he had first-hand knowledge of Nathan's circumstances and pain. Nathan icily clarified that Sebastian's relationship with his daughter was irrelevant to his own relationship with his son and thus was of zero interest to him. With the bearing and tone of an affronted professor, he pronounced the session over.

I suggest you float this exchange in the back of your mind as you make your way through the book. I'll be returning to it in the Epilogue, by which time you'll be well prepared for my take on why Sebastian's well-meaning empathic offering likely slammed into a brick wall and what you can do to avoid similar client reactions in your own sessions. But first, you have some reading, thinking, feeling, wondering, and experimenting to do.

1 THE INVENTION, EVOLUTION, AND DIFFERENTIATION OF EMPATHY

Empathy is empathizing; and we understand its constitution better by tracing its origins, developmental features, and specific functional uses.
—Anna Aragno, *The Language of Empathy* (2008, pp. 714-715)

Sharon and Graham had been married 35 years when Sharon died. A few weeks after the memorial service, their long-time friends Art and Carolyn flew into town to visit Graham in his home. Carolyn told me later that when he met them at the door, Graham was calm, if subdued. But then, as they walked with him into his living room, into the airless emptiness of Sharon's absence, raw grief broke through, and he started to sob. Art and Carolyn's eyes immediately welled with tears, and their hearts, heavy and aching with Graham's, filled with compassionate concern for his well-being.

Then, without warning, Carolyn was body slammed by the recognition that either she or Art would too soon be living the hell of exactly this scenario. She had, of course, always known and accepted that one of them would eventually lose the other. But in this moment, in Graham's presence, she wasn't contemplating an obvious fact as an abstract idea; she was living the electrical

---
https://doi.org/10.1037/0000472-002
Empathic Engagement in Clinical Practice, by D. Flemons
Copyright © 2026 by the American Psychological Association. All rights reserved.

shock of an existential truth: Whomever of them survives the death of the other will be, like Graham, rawly, inconsolably bereft. As this stark epiphany took hold, the quality of Carolyn's felt experience spun backward, transforming from the sympathetic resonance of *shared* grief to the private nightmare and self-consciously focused fear of anticipated *personal* grief.

Soon, though, Carolyn's emotional world lurched again as she turned her caring attention and compassionate concern back toward Graham. The refocusing didn't lessen the intensity of what she was experiencing, but it reestablished her sympathetic alignment with the two men, and it occasioned a shift in how she was relating to her charged feeling. She found herself wondering about and thus listening for the distinctive details of Graham's loss, no longer from the vantage of her relationship with Art but from within the context—the story—of Graham's history with Sharon. As Carolyn imagined what it was like to *be* Graham, her heightened affect became a valuable contribution to the imaginative process of virtually embodying and tangibly interpreting—empathically making sense of—his unfolding experience.

We commonly conceive of sympathy, compassion, and empathy as types of feelings. This conception isn't entirely wrong, but it is decidedly incomplete. All three involve some kind of bodily expression; however, each also establishes—and/or is established by enacting—a particular quality of relationship, a signature way of bridging the self–other divide. In so doing, each uniquely alters the boundary defining and encompassing a sense of self in contradistinction to some other—that is, in contradistinction to someone or something you consider to be distinct from you.

Thinking clearly about the respective relational qualities of empathy, sympathy, and compassion—about what each is and does—necessitates first getting a handle on the curious, relational properties of the self. Establishing this understanding now, right at the outset, will help everything that follows fit into place, like pieces in a jigsaw puzzle.

SELF AND OTHER

The sense of identity requires the existence of another by whom one is known.
—R. D. Laing, *The Divided Self* (1965, p. 139)

Your brain doesn't know where your body ends and the world begins. Instead, it approximates a continually shifting boundary.
—Lisa Feldman Barrett & Karen S. Quigley, *Interoception* (2021, p. 6)

We generally treat the defining boundary of the self as a settled fact, coinciding, more or less, with the physical dimensions of the body. This assumption is supported and reinforced when, for example, not dressed warmly enough on a cold winter walk, you mutter, "I am freezing!" This sense of your self as commensurate with your body comes into foreground focus whenever you feel up against something other that is surrounding you—a too-high or low temperature, a too-glaring light or an intimidating darkness, a swarm of people or insects. This body-based self-identity is also etched when something is coming at or facing off against you—an exam, a nemesis, a competitor.

But sometimes, your sense of self expands or extends beyond the physical border of your body. Perhaps you feel affronted when someone turns up their nose at your hat, your outfit, your perfume or cologne. Or you feel personally attacked when one of your creations—a short story, a painting, a musical composition—is criticized. Or, while driving on the highway, a truck in the next lane suddenly swerves, just missing your car, and you yell, "Watch out, you almost hit me!" At such times, your sense of self can become more inclusive, encompassing not only your body but also something you're wearing, something you've made or produced, something you're driving.

And then, sometimes, your sense of self comes into sharp relief *within* your body–mind, set apart from some distinguished part of the whole of you. This happens whenever you judge, positively or negatively, some aspect of "you" as either admirable or inadequate. You love or hate the sound of your voice or something about your physical appearance. You are delighted at how good a cold cloth feels on your forehead, or you feel victimized by a physical pain. You praise your excellent memory, or you worry that your depression is creeping back. You assess an idea that occurs to you as inspired or worthless. You feel pride at how hard you've been working or regret something you did in the past. Whenever you judge some distinguished part of your experience—how you sound or look, a body sensation, a feeling, a thought, an action—the defining boundary of what feels to be your self adjusts accordingly.

Despite the fact that our "predominant models of the mind are spatial ones" (Margulies, 1989, p. 135), the self isn't a concrete thing with a constant presence or spatial location (Ricard & Singer, 2017, Investigating the Self section), and it isn't some "central manager" running the show (Barrett, 2017a, p. 37). Rather, the self is a relationally emergent sensibility that self-referentially comes into foreground focus in contradistinction to whatever or whomever it is, at the moment, perceiving and marking as not-self or other. The boundary circumscribing the self is not a physical line—it is simply a difference, a contrast (Bateson, 1972/2000). This difference becomes more pronounced and, concomitantly, the boundary demarcating the self more definitively etched whenever you feel particularly at odds with something or someone that is not just different but disturbingly so—not just other, but alien.

When you first meet a new client, each of you is other to the other. And if the client is mandated to treatment, they may at first relate to you not just as the stranger you are but as an adversary, a threat. As long as the client is experiencing you as an outsider, they will be wise to keep their guard up, self-consciously defending a sense of self in contrast to you and carefully parsing whatever you do, say, and recommend. Such behaviors don't generally sit well with clinicians, who get impatient with what they perceive as resistance or noncompliance.

Empathy is a brilliant way of altering this dynamic. Through your empathic engagement with the client, they come to recognize you more as an insider than an outsider, which makes it safe for them to relax their efforts to hold you at arm's length and hold what you're offering at bay. Their caution and reluctance can give way to trust and a willingness to entertain possibilities for change. But empathy also occasions a shift in you. The more you give voice to your understanding of how the client is experiencing and making sense of their world, the less you will distinguish them as alien and their choices as irrational. This makes it easier for you to shift from urging compliance to inviting collaboration.

But I'm getting ahead of myself. A deep appreciation of how empathy works begins with a clear understanding of how the perception (and, correspondingly, the conception) of self and other changes in response to changes in the boundary separating them. The best way of illustrating this is to tell you the story about soup that I mentioned in the Introduction.

When my kids were young, my wife and I often took them to a nearby restaurant that featured a dish called "Two Soups in a Bowl." For a slight upcharge, you could ask for two of the four soups on the menu to be served in the same bowl. I always went with the ochre-colored tortilla and the green split pea. Because of the soups' comparable dense consistencies, the chef could simultaneously ladle each one into opposite sides of the bowl, and they would form a relatively straight diagonal line where they met during the filling—a discernable boundary between them.

One night, I told our waiter that I wanted to conduct an experiment. As my kids slunk down in their seats and rolled their eyes, I said I wanted to order "Two Soups in a Bowl" but wished to make a slight modification to the order. I'd like, I said, for my two soups to be split pea and, wait for it, split pea. I clarified that I would, of course, pay the added cost of having the dish prepared in the usual manner, but in exchange, I asked that he ensure that the chef did not cut corners and just do a single pour. He agreed. When he brought our meal to the table, the waiter confirmed that my bowl contained two separately and simultaneously ladled split-pea soups. I invited my wife and kids to join me in finding the boundary dividing them, but with the color and consistency of the distinct soups the same, none of us could locate it. The difference between the two soups was indifferentiated—there but undetectable.

Something analogous happens whenever the perceived difference (and thus the assumed boundary) between your sense of self and some not-self—something other—is indifferentiated. You can get a first-hand, visceral handle on this idea by taking a couple of minutes to experiment with what is commonly known as mindfulness meditation. When you get to the end of this paragraph, sit in a comfortable, upright posture and bring your attention to your breathing. It might help if you close your eyes. Don't purposefully alter the rate or depth of the breath. As best you can, allow its easy, automatic movement to continue while you bring your fully absorbed awareness in line with it. As you breathe in, know you're breathing in, and as you breathe out, know you're breathing out (Goldstein, 2016, p. 50), noticing the sounds and sensations associated with each. When your attention drifts, plucked away by a stray feeling, thought, or perception, you'll be lost for a little while. But when you realize, "Oh wait, I forgot to follow my breath," just notice the fact of the distraction and, without judging yourself, return to your breath. See you in a couple of minutes.

Welcome back. You may have noticed something interesting happening during the time, however brief, when your noticing remained closely aligned with your breathing. As the Zen teacher Shunryu Suzuki (2006) advised, "If you are concentrated on your breathing you will forget yourself, and if you forget yourself you will be concentrated on your breathing" (p. 139). Maintaining a close awareness of your breathing is different from thinking about it (or thinking about being aware of it). When you follow along with it, the content and pattern of your observing closely match the content and pattern of the breath being observed, so the difference, and thus the boundary, between awareness and breath—between observer and observed, between self and other—is minimized. Becoming absorbed in the process, you "forget about your self."

An interpersonal version of self–other boundary dissolution is experienced by people who sing together. Imagine standing in the midst of a bunch of people you don't know. As you look around, you notice individuals who differ from you (and each other) in age, culture, height, hair length and/or color, eye and/or skin color, dress, and/or language and accent. Surrounded by such a range of dissimilarities, your sense of self is distinctly defined in contradistinction. This will soon change if you've all been brought together as a choir to rehearse a song you've each individually learned. As the group moves through the tune in rhythmic and harmonic coordination, each person's voice melds and interweaves with those around it. In the process, the countless differences that distinguish each person as separate and unique—that distinguish you from the others—become mostly irrelevant for the duration of the song. During the singing, as insignificant differences become indifferentiated, the boundary demarcating your self-conscious, circumscribed self becomes indiscernible. A bunch of previously discrete selves coalesce as a group. "Ah," you think, "*we* sound good." Your group identity coheres still more in performance when you can hear the effect of standing in front of an audience: "Singing to *them*," you recognize, "is inspiring to *us*."

The mutually defining, interdependent polarity of self and other operates like, and often in conjunction with, the contrast between "us" and "them." What is encompassed within—included as part of—your definition of "self" or your grouping of "us" is in part both determining of and determined by what is excluded and thereby defined as "other" or "them." Both processes of complementary categorization—self/other and us/them—create, and/or are created by, the differences distinguishing who or what you are from who or what you're not. As Fischer (2013) put it, "There are no others apart from us, and there is no us apart from them" (p. 98).

Back in the 1980s, when my two brothers and I would return to our family home in Calgary, Canada, for a visit, friends of our parents who called the house could never tell which of us had answered the phone. Was it Tom? Douglas? Ward? For these family friends, my and my brothers' voices were so close in timbre and cadence they were impossible to tell apart.

Empathy, sympathy, and compassion have proved similarly difficult for theorists and researchers to distinguish clearly. So alike in so many respects, the three concepts have often eluded efforts to disentangle them consistently. Empathy? Sympathy? Compassion? Which of you is on the phone?

One year in the late 1980s, I came home for a family reunion. Inspired by the sonic similarities between my and my brothers' voices, possessed of a mischievous spirit, and aided by the fact that caller ID had not yet been invented, I made a quick call one late afternoon to Ward's wife at the time, Lori. I was hoping to prank her by successfully impersonating her husband. "Hey, Sweetheart, it's me," I said, "I'm just heading out. Need me to pick anything up on my way home?" I wasn't confident I could sustain my ruse for long, so I kept the call short and sweet. Lori replied lightly, "No, I'm good. See you soon." I couldn't tell if I had successfully hoodwinked her; later, she clarified that she'd been playing me. She possessed a better ear and—surprise, surprise—more familiarity than my parents' friends with Ward's voice, but she'd also had innumerable phone conversations with him, and this one stood out as different. I've always called people I care about "Sweetheart," but this was not an endearment my brother commonly used, so my idiosyncratic word choice drew attention to itself and gave me away. The words we use, the words we choose, matter (cf. Le Guin, 2004, p. 206). More on this a little later.

What follows is some confusion-prevention ear training designed to help you make sense of empathy, sympathy, and compassion so that you can, with Lori-like discernment, reliably tell them apart and keep them straight. Although they are intriguingly similar, each can be understood as a unique means of regarding, experiencing, and relating to someone or something on the other side of the self–other or us–them divide. The tell-tale differences I develop next are grounded, in part, in the three terms' respective etymologies, but, as you'll see, the contrasts extend outward from there, ramifying through their respective enactments.

DIFFERENTIATING EMPATHY, SYMPATHY, AND COMPASSION

Words tell the history of a concept: their meanings and etymologies are the factual story of a concept as much as any novel is the fictional story of its characters.

–Frederic William Lieber, *The Legacy of Empathy* (1995, p. 34)

Poets depend on etymological information in order to make hidden connections between apparently unrelated ideas and to establish metaphoric consonance in cases where a superficial reader might think the metaphoric thread has been broken.

–K. K. Ruthven, *The Poet as Etymologist* (1969, p. 10)

Strike a tuning fork that has been precision engineered to vibrate at 440 beats per second, and it will produce a clear tone that, if you're a musician with perfect pitch, you'll recognize as "concert pitch"—the A above middle C. This particular note—A440—is a common reference point for orchestras.[1] Before the conductor comes out on stage, the principal oboist

---

[1] Some orchestras use an ever so slightly "sharper" note—an A442 or A444—to achieve a brighter sound, but that's another story.

plays concert pitch, which each of the other musicians uses to calibrate the tuning of their instrument to match all the others precisely. Thanks to this communal adjustment, the audience can enjoy everyone playing together "in tune." The frequencies align.

Now, if you place two such tuning forks next to each other and strike just one of them, the second one will vibrate along with the first, producing that same A. Similarly, if you bow one of the open strings on a violin (G, D, A, or E), the resulting sound waves will cause the corresponding string on a nearby violin to vibrate along with it, producing the same note. Engineers call this phenomenon *sympathetic resonance*. The word "sympathy" comes from the Greek roots *syn* ("together") and *pathos* ("suffering" or "feeling"). Combined, they form the idea of "suffering with," "feeling with," or "feeling together." Tuning forks and violins vibrate together in sympathy, and sometimes, so to speak, do people. Indeed, the Scottish philosopher David Hume used the analogy of a violin's strings resonating with other strings to describe how we resonate with others' pains and pleasures as if they were our own (Jinpa, 2015, p. 9).

At the beginning of the chapter, I told you what happened when Graham, recently bereaved, entered his living room with his friends. The moment he started to register the loss of his wife, as his grief came over him, Art and Carolyn were right there with him. Their tears welled up. The three of them were in instant affective accord, instant sympathetic resonance, before any words were spoken or conscious thoughts were formed. I say more about this human version of sympathetic resonance a little later.

Many authors have undertaken reasoned arguments, thought experiments, and well-designed studies to tease out how and why such sympathetic responses occur. Others have explored the same questions about related phenomena, namely compassion and, particularly, empathy. But exactly how are they related? It all depends on whom you ask. Throughout the literature, sympathy and empathy are often confused (Clark, 2010; Wispé, 1986). Daniel Batson (2009) found that "with remarkable consistency exactly the same state that some scholars have labeled empathy others have labeled sympathy," and he could "discern . . . no clear basis—either historical or logical—for favoring one labeling scheme over another" (p. 8; see also Cuff et al., 2016). Batson himself, who has devoted much of his career to thoroughly illuminating the nature of what he calls "empathic concern," used neither history nor logic to guide his choice of that term. He "settled on [it] in the 1970s when *sympathy* seemed patronizing and *compassion* carried connotations of religion" (Batson, 2023, p. 12).

Batson (2009) pointed out that although authors "typically agree that empathy is important, they often disagree about why it is important, about what effects it has, about where it comes from, and even about what it is" (p. 3). The different conceptualizations are at least partly a reflection of "distinct psychological processes that vary, sometimes widely, in their function, phenomenology, mechanisms, and effects" (Coplan, 2011b, p. 42). Clearly, "opportunities for disagreement abound" (Batson, 2009, p. 3), which has resulted in "almost as many definitions of empathy as there are researchers in the field" (Singer & Lamm, 2009, p. 82), indeed, "almost as many definitions as there are people who use the word" (Alda, 2021, 16:25).

Empathy has been conceived of as a "way of being" and "a process rather than a state" (Rogers, 2007, p. 2), as "a tool, a skill, a kind of communication, a listening stance, a type of introspection, a capacity, a power, a form of perception or observation, a disposition, . . . a feeling" (Basch, 1983, p. 102), as well as "emotional resonance or contagion, motor mimicry, a complex cognitive and imaginative capacity, perspective taking, kinesthetic modeling, a firing of mirror neurons, [and] concern for others" (Lanzoni, 2018, p. 3). Whew! As Alice, in Lewis Carroll's (1872/2009) *Through the Looking Glass*, said, "That's a great deal to make one word mean" (p. 152). When Humpty Dumpty would "make a word do a lot of work like that," he would "always pay it extra" (Carroll, 1872/2009, p. 152). If we were to adopt Humpty Dumpty's reimbursement policy, we'd owe "empathy" a fortune. Definitional and conceptual variation has been a characteristic feature of the word since it was first introduced. Alice wondered aloud to Humpty Dumpty "whether you *can* make words mean so many different things" (Carroll, 1872/2009, p. 151). Clearly, you can because, when it comes to empathy, we have, though not without constructing something of a Tower of Babel.

Current empathy experts hail from far-ranging disciplines: history, philosophy (of ethics, aesthetics, phenomenology, and hermeneutics), anthropology, communication, ethology, theology, neuroscience, political science, sociology, organizational psychology, personality psychology, social psychology, developmental psychology, medicine (both physicians and nurses), and psychotherapy (psychologists, psychiatrists, psychoanalysts, counselors, social workers, and family therapists). The result of such rich diversity has been a field marked less by synergy than cacophony and less by cross-fertilization than crosstalk. Different authors, even within the same discipline, have pursued what amounts to parallel or even incompatible lines of inquiry, talking past each other in a way that recalls the overlapping dialogue so characteristic of Aaron Sorkin TV shows and movies, such as *A Few Good Men*, *The West Wing*, and *The Social Network*. Martin Buber would have called such exchanges between Sorkin characters on a screen or among empathy experts in articles and books "monologue disguised as dialogue" (Cissna & Anderson, 2002, p. 52).

If there's no consensus on an understanding or definition of empathy and no consensus about how to achieve consensus (or at least some kind of inter-writer reliability), every contributor to the literature risks coming across like a Humpty Dumpty impersonator. Perhaps you remember in *Through the Looking Glass* when "in rather a scornful tone," Humpty Dumpty said to Alice, "'When I use a word, . . . it means just what I choose it to mean—neither more nor less'" (Carroll, 1872/2009, p. 151). Such an imperious approach can offer you, as a reader, the possibility of developing a degree of ideational clarity inside the cloistered culture and vernacular of whatever study, article, chapter, or book you're currently visiting. However, without some kind of Concept and Terminology edition of Google Translate in your pocket, you're faced with starting from scratch when you visit the next one.

Most authors accept that there is no final authority, no objective arbiter of meaning who can pronounce one definition superior to another (e.g., Batson, 2023, p. 57; Eisenberg et al., 1991, p. 64). If, as de Saussure (1916/1987) claimed, there is a fundamental disconnect between signifier and signified, between word and concept, then one definition of empathy is as valid as the next (see Ruthven, 1969, p. 12, who traces such a position back to Hermogenes in Plato's *Cratylus*). And the reverse is also true—given a well-defined concept, the question of what label to affix to it—empathy, sympathy, or compassion—becomes moot and thus trivial. This is certainly Paul Bloom's (2016) position: "I *hate* terminological arguments," he said, "nothing important rests on the specific words we use so long as we understand one another" (p. 40). Batson (2023) similarly concluded that "as long as it's clear that we're talking about the same . . . emotional state, then to use a different label is fine" (p. 12). A lovesick, 15-year-old girl in Act II, Scene II of *Romeo and Juliet* (Shakespeare, 1599/2011) put it this way: "What's in a name? That which we call a rose/ By any other name would smell as sweet; So Romeo would, were he not Romeo call'd, Retain that dear perfection which he owes/Without that title" (2.2.43–47).

Sure. And yet labeling isn't a one-way street: "Words . . . have what A. S. Palmer called 'the Parthian power . . . of shooting backwards . . . and controlling the ideas which they are supposed only to express'" (Ruthven, 1969, p. 35). Would Romeo "retain that dear perfection" (Shakespeare, 1599/2011, 2.2.46) if he were to "take [Juliet] at [her] word" and "be new baptized" (2.2.49b–50) as "Mikey"? And would the "light through yonder window" breaking be as dazzling as the sun (2.2.2–3) if the young woman declaiming her love were named "Gertie"? Would you take a tragedy entitled *Mikey and Gertie* seriously? I probably wouldn't, either.

As I said earlier, words matter. Names and labels make a difference (Barrett & Russell, 1998, pp. 979–980), but so do prepositions, including those that operate inside words, embedded as prefixes.

When you label a concept, process, or phenomenon, you classify it as a something, etching a boundary that sets it apart from what it isn't and establishing relationships between it and other somethings that, in various ways, it resembles. This means that the name isn't a stand-alone blank slate, even when freshly coined. Whether established, borrowed, or invented, it comes with a quality of sound ("Romeo" vs. "Mikey"; "Juliet" vs. "Gertie"), with associations, and with a history, if only its etymology, that contribute to the larger context of its meaning. And in the process of defining it, you place it within a network of understandings and assumptions, some stated, some implicit, that shape what you make of it—and what you can make with it.

Which brings us back to the term *empathy*. When it first appeared on the scene in English and American psychology circles at the beginning of the 20th century, it wasn't springing fresh and fully formed from Athena's head (though Greece, or at least the Greek language, had a role in its origin story—I get to that in a minute). It was, in fact, a translation of a German word and concept—*Einfühlung*—that had been knocking about Europe since the 18th century.

EINFÜHLUNG: THE ORIGINS OF "EMPATHY" IN GERMAN PHILOSOPHY

Many authors assume that the philosopher and psychologist Theodor Lipps invented the word Einfühlung, but although he did much to promulgate it and refine its meaning, the art historian Robert Vischer is the one who is more accurately credited with coining it, in 1873, in a dissertation on aesthetics. Wanting to "convert abstract principles of aesthetic philosophy into sensory and motor processes" (Lieber, 1995, p. 168), Vischer wrote about coming to know a work of art through Einfühlung—through a process of "feeling one's way into" it. For him, aesthetic appreciation involved projecting the self into an object of beauty (Jahoda, 2005, p. 154).

However, the story doesn't end there. Or, better put, the history of the word doesn't start there. When Vischer came up with the word Einfühlung, he perhaps wasn't aware that 100 years earlier, the German philosopher Johann Gottfried von Herder (1744–1803) was using the same and related terms to refer to "knowledge that was sensory in origin with emphasis on the senses operating all at once and holistically" (Edwards, 2013, p. 271). Herder broke "down the rigid division between subject and object by realizing that everything is interconnected and works together . . . by virtue of . . . [the] oneness of the whole" (Meinecke, 1936/1972, as cited in Edwards, 2013, p. 272). For example, rather than judging other cultures from the outside, Herder sought

> to penetrate—"feel himself" (*Einfühlen* is his invention, a hundred years before Lipps or Dilthey or Croce)—into their essence, grasp what it must be like to live, contemplate goals, act and react, think, imagine, in the unique ways dictated by their circumstances, and so grasp the patterns of [their] life. (Berlin, 1976, p. 173, italic in original)

Herder insisted that "one must enter the time, the place, the entire history [of a people]"; one must "feel oneself [*sich einfülen*] into everything" (Berlin, 1976, p. 186, italic in original).

For both Herder and Vischer, Einfühlung was a method of sensory, affective, and imaginative knowing that provided a means for crossing the boundary separating subject from object, self from other. For Vischer, it was the result of a form of "bodily mimicry" or "inner imitation" (Pigman, 1995, p. 240).

Theodor Lipps then came along at the turn of the 20th century and described such knowing as a blending of self and other (Edwards, 2013, p. 276), a fusing of the observer and the object as a result of the difference between them becoming irrelevant: "The contrast between myself and the object disappears" (Lipps, 1903a, as cited in Jahoda, 2005, p. 154). By way of illustration, he described himself observing a tightrope walker: "I am, according to my direct (unmediated) awareness in him; I am there high up. I am transported there. Not next to the acrobat, but exactly within him, where he is. This is thus the full meaning of '*Einfühlung*'" (as cited in Lanzoni, 2018, p. 33, italic in original).

About the same time, various authors were casting about for the best way to render the conceptual nuances of Einfühlung into English. In 1895, the English novelist Vernon Lee (aka Violet Paget) suggested the word "sympathy" (Wispé, 1987, p. 18). A committee of philosophers offered "aesthetic sympathy"; others suggested "animation" or "semblance" (Lanzoni, 2018, p. 9). None quite landed or took hold. But then, in 1908, the psychologist Edward Titchener, whose interest in etymology was matched by his considerable knowledge of Latin and Greek, came up with "empathy," a neologism modeled on the Greek roots of "sympathy" (*sym* "with" and *pathos* "suffering" or "feeling," which together mean "suffering or feeling with") and inspired by the German roots of Einfühlung ("feeling in" or "feeling into"). Whereas *sympathy* had to do with "feeling *with*" the other, *empathy* (combining *en*, "in," and *pathos*, "suffering" or "feeling") was concerned with "feeling *into*" the other (see Wispé, 1987, p. 21).[2] The difference between the two terms turns entirely on the prepositions that form part of their respective etymologies.

Prepositions establish spatial, temporal, or conceptual relationships, specifying the location or understanding of one thing in relation to another. To say that Little Red Riding Hood is *with* her grandmother is different from saying she is *in* her grandmother. Damn wolf. Likewise, to say that you are feeling *with* your client—alongside them, sharing their pain—is different from saying that you are feeling or sensing your way *into* their experience. As I talk about in Chapter 2, feeling something together *with* another person establishes a quality of companionship and a shared sense of *us*. Such mutuality strengthens personal bonds; however, it undermines professional relationships. Clients need to be able to lose their composure or their temper, trusting that you will keep yours. That can't happen if you are with them in their suffering. In Chapter 3, I offer suggestions for how to safely and effectively stay collected in challenging circumstances, but the capacity to do so begins here, with a seemingly small prepositional shift. You commit not to sharing the client's experience but to understanding it, and you accomplish that by projecting your imagination into it.

EMPATHY: FEELING *INTO*

It could be argued that one [does] not really understand a word until one [has] grasped its root and considered its relations to other words with the same root.
—Walter Kaufmann, in Martin Buber's *I and Thou* (1923/1970, p. 33)

Empathy [is] a penetration, a kind of travel. . . . You enter another person's pain as you'd enter another country, through immigration and customs, border crossing by way of query: What grows where you are? What are the laws? What animals graze here?
—Leslie Jamison, *The Empathy Exams* (2014)

Most contemporary definitions of empathy, save for some in philosophy, don't acknowledge or incorporate the original notion of it having to do with

---

[2]That same year, the psychologist James Ward proposed the same translation; it isn't known whether he and Titchener, who were both contributing editors to the journal *Mind*, had conferred or not (Lanzoni, 2018, pp. 50–51).

"aesthetic projection" (Batson, 2009). Perhaps authors don't know about its etymology or consider it irrelevant, or perhaps they hold to the idea that a proper definition should be informed by research results rather than historical precedent, that a definition should be, as Hallenbeck (1981) argued, "psychological rather than lexicological" (p. 226).

Regardless of whether the lacuna reflects a lack of awareness or a considered disregard, it represents a missed opportunity for conceptual clarity, given that the word *empathy* wouldn't exist at all if not for its etymology. In coining *empathy*, Titchener succeeded in fashioning a translation of Einfühlung that retained something of the original's sense of coming to know the other from within. Rather than projecting the imagination to an outside vantage in search of a detached, disembodied judgment of the other, Einfühlung—empathy— involves projecting the imagination into the other in search of an embodied, contextually rich sensibility.

Ignoring this provenance drains empathy of its evocative richness, rendering it a pallid synonym of *sympathy*. It also obscures the sense of empathy as a purposeful crossing of the self–other divide. When empathy is considered only to be something individually felt rather than recognized as a process interactively undertaken, it makes it more likely that its relational core will get lost in the shuffle, that it will be misconstrued as a localized trait the self has (something the self possesses) or a localized state the self enters (something the self feels).

As a clinician and supervisor, I am primarily concerned with how therapists and other professionals can best employ empathy in conversations with clients. Indeed, most of the rest of the book is devoted to delineating and demonstrating the skills involved in this means of engagement. But first, I need to say more about what makes empathy distinct from and similar to other related ways of crossing the self–other divide, particularly sympathy and compassion. In so doing, I'll have the opportunity to address another issue that has hovered over the field—the question of how broad or narrow a definition of empathy should be. Preston and de Waal (2002) advocated for an inclusive, big-tent approach, one that could take "different views . . . and cohere [them] into a unified whole" (p. 3), producing a definition relevant "across disciplines, situations, and species" (Coplan, 2011a, p. 5). Others have headed in the opposite direction, arguing for the importance of small-tent definitions: "We need more specificity," Coplan said, "not more generality" (p. 5).

To avoid confusion and the Aaron Sorkin effect, we require a detailed accounting of what empathy entails, and this necessity can't be satisfied by one inclusive, all-encompassing definition. But this means "we need to refine our conceptual framework of empathy so as to distinguish clearly several related processes that too often get confused, conflated, or ignored" (Coplan, 2011b, p. 44). That is, we can satisfy the need for specificity and address Preston and de Waal's (2002) call for linking together wide-ranging research interests and results by introducing a *net* of closely defined and interconnected terms and concepts. What's needed is "a theoretical framework that makes salient the relevant differences and similarities between the multiple processes that get referred to as empathy" (Coplan, 2011b, p. 44).

In staking a claim for his definition of "empathic concern," Batson (2023, p. 3) advised readers who prefer a different term for this concept to make a mental substitution as they read, replacing Batson's term with their own. Here, I reverse the direction of and responsibility for such translating. Rather than leaving it up to you to substitute your own or others' labels for mine, I make the switch myself and then reference the term the author used. This practice is in accord with those writers (e.g., Fleischacker, 2019; Prinz, 2011) who, for example, talk about Adam Smith's and/or David Hume's ideas about empathy, despite the fact that Hume and Smith were using the word "sympathy" to convey an empathic sensibility long before the word "empathy" had been invented (in, e.g., Hume's [1739] *A Treatise of Human Nature* and A. Smith's [1759] *A Theory of Moral Sentiments*).

A last orienting comment before we embark: Because I consider empathy and related terms to be descriptive of unique patterns of relationship between self and other, the definitions I offer specify the nature of the relationship each establishes, as well as its effect on the self–other divide. The following descriptions will become prescriptions, or at least recommendations, in subsequent chapters for how best to put empathy into practice in clinical settings. Let's start with "sympathy".

SYMPATHY: FEELING *WITH*

The sun had not yet risen. The sea was indistinguishable from the sky, except that the sea was slightly creased as if a cloth had wrinkles in it. Gradually as the sky whitened a dark line lay on the horizon dividing the sea from the sky and the grey cloth became barred with thick strokes moving, one after another.

–Virginia Woolf, *The Waves* (1931)

At the beginning of the chapter, I told you about Art's and Carolyn's eyes immediately brimming with tears when their friend Graham began to cry. Researchers would classify this as an instance of emotional contagion, "whereby a person automatically mimics someone's facial expression, resulting in a weaker version of the same emotion as that of the person being mimicked" (van Baaren et al., 2009, p. 32). In 1992, scientists studying macaques identified what they later came to call *mirror neurons*—brain cells in the ventral premotor cortex that fired regardless of whether a monkey was grasping something or was merely observing the grasping (di Pellegrino et al., 1992). Subsequent research has identified other regions of the brain (including those associated with emotion, such as the insula and amygdala) where mirror neurons and brain systems with mirroring properties are active, not only in monkeys but also in humans (Debes, 2017, p. 55). There is mounting evidence that these mirroring properties of human brains have an important role in emotional contagion, but this role is neither fully understood (Paz et al., 2022) nor fully documented (van Baaren et al., 2009, p. 32). Batson (2023, p. 47) cited various studies that question the degree to which mirroring is unlearned and automatic.

Regardless of the neurological substrate of the mirroring, sympathy involves a quality of the resonance I mentioned earlier. When I feel with what you're feeling, your feelings and mine resonate. The early American psychologist James Mark Baldwin described the result this way: "The external and indeed the internal boundaries between you and me are swept away, and I feel your calamity really as my own" (as cited in Wispé, 1986, p. 315).

Sympathetic Resonance

Paul Bloom (2016) made a splash when he proclaimed in the title of a book that he is, in the words of Jesse Prinz (2011), "against empathy."[3] Underscoring that empathy is deeply flawed when relied on as a means for guiding moral decisions or responsible actions, he explained that "it grounds foolish judgments and often motivates indifference and cruelty. It can . . . corrode certain important relationships, such as between a doctor and a patient, and make us worse at being friends, parents, husbands, and wives" (Bloom, 2016, pp. 2–3). He cautioned parents, for example, against "absorb[ing] the . . . suffering" of their children, noting how unhelpful it would be to panic "along with" a "teenager who is panicked because she left her homework to the last minute" (Bloom & Zaki, 2016, para. 7). Excellent point. However, in terms of the network of terms I'm defining here, the phenomenon of sharing "an emotion . . . with another" (Prinz, 2011, p. 230), of "feeling what

---

[3]The philosopher Peter Goldie (2011) has also staked out an antiempathy position. Not surprisingly, given the widely divergent definitions and considerations of empathy suffusing the field, Goldie's empathy antipathy, having to do with a particular kind of perspective-shifting, is different from Bloom's and Prinz's moral-action concerns.

others feel" (Bloom, 2016, p. 130), is better understood not as empathy but as *sympathetic resonance* (cf. Basch, 1990, p. 3, who refers to "affective resonance").

Such resonance has been extensively studied, most commonly under the guise of terms such as "empathy,"[4] "emotional empathy," "emotional contagion," or "empathic distress." Neuroscientists working in this area cite growing evidence that, when it comes to affect, given the right conditions, what's yours is (or at least can become) mine (Zaki, 2019, p. 14). Or what's yours can become ours (Paz et al., 2022).

> Changes in one person's body often prompt changes in another person's body, whether the two are romantically involved, just friends, or strangers meeting for the first time. When you're with someone you care about, your breathing can synchronize, as can the beating of your hearts, whether you're in casual conversation or a heated argument. . . . We often mirror each other's movements in a dance that neither of us is aware of and that is choreographed by our brains. One of us leads, the other follows, and sometimes we switch. (Barrett, 2020, p. 84)

My brain represents your pain in much the same way it represents my own. Although the relationship between physiological and sympathetic pain is complex (e.g., Zaki et al., 2016), researchers have found that the same brain regions—particularly the anterior insula and the middle anterior cingulate cortex (Kanske et al., 2015)—become activated by both "firsthand experience and the vicarious experience of sensations or emotions experienced by another person" (Bernhardt & Singer, 2012, p. 15). This overlap holds true for both pain (Decety & Lamm, 2009, pp. 199–200; Lamm et al., 2011) and, at least partially (Batson, 2023, p. 47), for nonpain affective states (Timmers et al., 2018).

Most studies on emotional contagion focus on what gets picked up and shared through sight. Your face and body are activated by and synchronize with what you see in the face and body of the person in front of you, which prompts a syncing up of neuronal firing and emotional states (Paz et al., 2022, p. 9). But contagion can also be initiated through hearing and smell (Maibom, 2022, p. 114). For example, the chemical composition of anxious sweat differs from exercise sweat, and this difference can be nonconsciously perceived and responded to by those who smell it.

---

[4]Feeling the same distress as another has been called empathy not only by Bloom (2016) but, as Batson (2023, p. 11) noted, also by Decety and Lamm (2009), de Vignemont and Singer (2006), and Eisenberg and Strayer (1987, p. 5).

In the 1970s, Karla McLaren introduced the word *empath* into the American pop-culture lexicon to denote people who are "exceptionally sensitive to the emotions, circumstances, and needs of everyone and everything around them" (McLaren, 2013, p. 4). She described what it was like for her as a young person to possess this capacity:

> My intense . . . receptivity made me feel as if I were on fire with the emotions of others. I picked up so many emotions and so much non-verbal social information from everyone around me that I often didn't know who I was or what I felt. (McLaren, 2013, p. 5)

I would rebrand such interpersonally sensitive people as *sympaths*, given that the boundary demarcating their sense of self isn't distinguished when they're in sympathetic resonance with those around them. Recall that when two ladles of the same kind of soup are poured separately into a bowl, the difference between them—and thus the boundary separating them—doesn't show up. It is indiscernible. Similarly, if you are feeling strongly about something—whether negative or positive—and I, in response to you, share your feeling, the countless differences between us become, for the time being, mostly unremarkable and irrelevant for both of us. The boundaries demarcating our respective senses of self are diffused by our shared affect and the accompanying communal sense of us.

But then, if, in the midst of the blurred identities of our resonance, our communality, I find myself feeling bad for you and/or becoming concerned about you,[5] it introduces a difference, a discontinuity, between us. An ever-so-slight shift in my relationship to you—from feeling *with* you to caring *about* your well-being—establishes a demarcated vantage from which to consider you. In the act of turning toward you, I subtly set myself apart, and I'm no longer to the same degree swept up in your—indeed, in what had become our—experience. Like a dark line forming on the horizon between dark sea and dark sky, an interstitial furrow insinuates itself between self and other.

An analog to this phenomenon can be found in the practice of mindfulness meditation. In everyday, nonmeditative awareness, we get buffeted by and caught up in unbidden moods or feelings and/or with unbidden trains or flurries of thoughts, images, sensations, perceptions, memories, and anticipations. We are so often in the thrall of—in sympathetic resonance with—whatever is visited on us that we become defined by it. Such inner weather tacitly contextualizes and thus demonstrably determines our sense of and response to ourselves and the world.

---

[5]Maibom (2017) noted that "sadness for . . . [the other] tends to morph into a concern for" them (p. 27): The two go hand in hand.

However, just as in the meditation experiment you carried out earlier, where you followed your breath in the cycling of inhales and exhales, you can position and ready your awareness to turn toward, recognize, and acknowledge whatever rises within you. In so doing, you introduce a discrete discontinuity in the relationship between your observing and your unbidden experience. With practice and intention, you can reposition your awareness, at least for fleeting moments, so that it is situated just beside your experience rather than caught up and defined by it. This allows you to *have* thoughts and emotions rather than simply *be* them (see Jinpa, 2015, p. 95).

The unintentional, interpersonal version of this shift in relationship plays out in situations where sympathetic resonance holds sway, such as in what happened to Carolyn in Graham's living room. When the welling up of her tears was followed by a welling up of sadness and concern (feeling bad for Graham and worried about him)—a slight crease was introduced into the automatic mirroring of Graham's distress. Within the dissolved boundaries of their resonance, Carolyn's caring about Graham both drew her to him and distinguished a sense of self somewhat apart from him. This is the shape of *sympathetic concern*, an essential protective factor for people working in the helping professions. The commitment to caring *about* and being concerned *for* the well-being of your clients introduces and maintains an identity-defining line of demarcation between you and them, which buffers the sympathetic resonance you feel *with* them.

Sympathetic Concern

Batson (2023, p. 212) clearly distinguished between sympathetic *resonance* (feeling as another feels) and sympathetic (what he terms empathic) *concern*, which, like compassion (p. 50), involves feeling *for* another. Sympathetic concern is other-oriented but not alien-oriented. That is, although it involves outward-focused caring, it does not extend to those we dismiss as beyond the pale (cf. Kongtrul, 2016). We feel sympathetic concern especially for people who are important to us (Jinpa, 2015, pp. 113–114), for those with whom we already feel close (Goubert et al., 2009, p. 160) or for those with whom we resonate as co-contributors of a defining sense of us— family, friends, and meaningful communities, whether religious, political, academic, recreational, or physical. Such privileging of ingroups (Gutsell & Inzlicht, 2010) is one of the main reasons Bloom (2016) leveled criticism at what I identify as "sympathy" (which he calls empathy). There is evidence, albeit mixed (Batson, 2023, p. 215), that sympathetic concern tends to be limited to "those who are close to us, those who are similar to us, and those we see as more attractive or vulnerable and less scary" (Bloom, 2016, p. 31).

Let's say you just heard that a loved one has been hospitalized following a car accident. Before you even see or talk to them, you'll likely be swept up in what might best be termed *empathy-inflected sympathy*—feeling sympathetic resonance with another by imagining their experience.[6] As I discuss later, full-on empathy is distinguishable from this in terms of intention and creation. With a commitment to knowing, empathy is a method for developing an embodied, context-rich *understanding* of the other. In contrast, empathy-inflected sympathy, though sparked by your empathic imagination, results in an experience of *shared feeling*—that is, with sympathetic resonance. As Klimecki and Singer (2012) noted, "observing or even simply imagining another person's affective state triggers an isomorphic affective response" (p. 370).

In addition to feeling *with* your loved one, you will immediately also feel bad *for* them, agonizing as you imagine the fear and pain they must have experienced during the accident and now are enduring in the hospital. Such a shared and caring passion typically reflects a tacit assumption that the person suffering is a victim of circumstance, of fate: Something bad—unfair, even—has happened *to* them (cf. Nussbaum, 2001, in reference to what she conceives of as compassion). You feel sympathy for those you deem to be unfairly afflicted, for those, in your estimation, who are vulnerable (Batson, 2023; Bloom, 2016; R. Epstein, 2017, p. 127), who lack guile and agency.

This heartfelt response will likely shift if, much to your dismay, you now learn that your loved one had been intoxicated when their car jumped the median and slammed into an oncoming truck. By viewing them no longer as a hapless victim but as the reckless perpetrator of their misfortune, judgment enters the picture, which tempers, alters, and/or complexifies your connection with them. "It's your own damn fault!" you can imagine exclaiming when you first visit them in the hospital. Sympathy wanes, slips away, or morphs into pity when you blame or otherwise consider the other to be alien (cf. R. D. Siegel & Germer, 2012, p. 15).

Pity is a desiccated form of sympathetic concern, what Buddhists would describe as the "near enemy" of compassion (Jinpa, 2015, p. 72). Although it involves an empathy-inflected turning toward the other, acknowledging their suffering in the face of their circumstances, pity distances the other as alien, inscribing a hard-and-fast distinguishing boundary that fully insulates against sympathetic resonance. When the other's plight grabs your attention

---

[6]Here the focus is on a painful experience, but if the other were to be celebrating joyful news, your empathy-inflected sympathy would reflect that reality. You'd be delighted with and for them.

without pulling your heartstrings, you feel sorry *for* them without identifying *with* them: Your sense of *us*—and your inclination to care—does not extend far enough to include them. Thus, regardless of what you see, you aren't moved by it much. Such hollowed-out sympathy is often plated with a side order of condescension (cf. Pence, 1983, p. 189). Instead of a tender embrace for someone you identify within an inclusive sense of us, you offer a curt, supercilious nod from across the self–other divide.

If at some point you were to decide that your loved one was a victim of their addiction and/or undermined by personal or developmental limitations (cf. Maibom, 2022, p. 93), the accusatory pointing of your index finger would relax, the division between the two of you would diminish, and you'd once again find it possible to feel bad with and tender toward them (cf. Batson, 2023, p. 211). By diminishing your sense of their culpability and thereby expanding your sense of *us* to include them, your sympathetic resonance and concern would be back in play.

Personal Distress

Emotional contagion has to do with sympathetic resonance. Because your "nervous system is bound up with the behavior of other humans" (Barrett, 2020, p. 91), when someone you care about is suffering, you'll tend to suffer alongside them, resonating with the felt sense (Gendlin, 1981, p. 32) of their struggle. Your shared visceral experience alters your perception of the differences—and thus the boundaries—between the two of you, diminishing your circumscribed sense of self, which, in turn, inscribes a mutual sense of us and prompts concern for the other's well-being.

This was certainly Carolyn's initial experience in Graham's living room. But then, in the midst of her sympathetic reaction to Graham's grief, she was deeply shaken by the realization that the future was staring her down. When death came for her or Art, the surviving partner was going to be as raw, lost, and inconsolable as Graham. The distress she'd been feeling with and for her friend doubled back on itself, becoming deeply personal and thus internally, rather than externally, focused. Initially connecting Carolyn and Graham, the suffering now came between them, etching the defining boundary of Carolyn's separate, despairing self (cf. Decety & Lamm, 2009; Eisenberg & Eggum, 2009).

Coplan (2011b) reported a difference in "the neural implementation of other-oriented perspective taking" and "self-oriented perspective taking" (p. 55), a difference that can be observed behaviorally. Researchers have demonstrated that if you imagine yourself parachuted into the circumstances faced by another (what they call an "imagine-self" scenario), you're more likely to get overwhelmed and emotionally (and perhaps physically) withdraw or retreat than if you leave your sense of self out of the equation and simply stay focused on the other's emotional and behavioral reactions to the circumstances (an "imagine-other" scenario) or, alternatively, do your best to remain "objective" (Batson, 2023; Batson et al., 1997; Decety & Lamm, 2009).

As I discuss later, these findings have significant implications for the practice of empathy. Becoming self-consciously self-concerned in the midst of sympathetic resonance or empathic exploration occasions a gestalt shift: Your imagined suffering becomes foreground; the other's actual suffering, background. Struggling to manage your experience, you no longer have the capacity to stay concerned or maintain a desire to help (cf. Eisenberg & Eggum, 2009).

For many years, I supervised family therapy graduate students in a training clinic attached to the university program in which I taught. The supervision was live, which meant I could see (from behind a one-way mirror) sessions unfolding in real time. I remember a particular evening, watching while one of my students, Marlene, struggled to connect with a challenging family (see Flemons, 2002, pp. 47–49, for a fuller description of the case). When they weren't loudly arguing and hurling accusations at each other, they were recounting gut-wrenching stories of the terror they had endured at the hands of the father, who had recently been imprisoned for domestic violence. The aftereffects of his beatings and threats were on full display in the mother and children's expressions of distrust, despair, and paralyzing fear. The more they described and displayed their pain, the more reserved and polite Marlene became.

After the family left, Marlene and I met for a postsession consultation. She was dismayed, she said, by all the damage the father's abuse had caused and said she couldn't imagine how the family would ever recover. "You feel bad for them?" I asked.

MARLENE: Just terrible. The whole situation is just so sad.

DOUGLAS: How do you anticipate that influencing your work with them?

Marlene said she believed compassion to be essential for good therapy. I agreed but suggested that her engagement with the family (it was really a disengagement from them) had more the trappings, the chilliness, of pity.

DOUGLAS: It was emotionally intense in there.

MARLENE: Tell me about it. It was overwhelming.

DOUGLAS: You were very polite to them.

MARLENE: I tried to be.

DOUGLAS: The thing is, they are particularly unruly, so your politeness created quite a contrast, perhaps giving them the impression that you'd written them off, like you'd already given up on them.

MARLENE: I didn't know what to do.

DOUGLAS: It's hard not to feel helpless if you see them as hopeless.

MARLENE: They're still reeling.

DOUGLAS: To move from pity to compassion, you'd need to connect with them, which would mean finding a different way to manage feeling overwhelmed. And that will be easier if you shift from seeing and treating the kids and the mother as broken to recognizing and acknowledging the vitality and life-affirming defiance at the heart of their commotion.

This became the focus of the next several sessions—Marlene learning how to engage compassionately and recognize and respond to the family's ways of being as indicators of strength and resilience. (In Chapter 3, I offer therapist self-care ideas and practices that, if it hadn't taken me so long to develop, Marlene could have used; in Chapter 5, I elaborate on the skill of empathically framing or categorizing client experiences in resourceful terms.)

COMPASSION: SUFFERING *TOGETHER*

Compassion . . . does not happen to a single individual in isolation, but as a response to another. It is a . . . reorientation that softens our sense of our individuality by bringing it into a felt relationship with the pain and needs of some other.

—Anne Harrington, A Science of Compassion or a Compassionate Science? (2002, p. 21)

Compassion is sympathy's etymological doppelgänger and its connotative and experiential complement. The Latin roots of *compassion* and the Greek roots of *sympathy* align in conveying the notion of shared suffering, of suffering (*pati/pathos*) together (*com/sym*). But whereas sympathy sweeps you up in an automatic mirroring of the affective experience of the other, compassion can be intentionally nurtured and developed (R. Epstein, 2017, p. 129). It involves a "willingness to feel pain with another, to feel another's pain as . . . [your] own" (Fischer, 2013, p. 32). However, as I discuss next, a compassionate *willingness*—a nonfearful openness—to feel pain doesn't necessarily mean you must or will feel the same as the other, particularly if you are skilled in compassionate meditation practices (Houshmand et al., 2002; Klimecki et al., 2013; Kongtrul, 2016). Compassion is a willingness to be resourcefully, affectively available to the other.

There are two other important differences. First, whereas sympathy most reliably shows up and takes hold when the other is someone you identify with or care about, compassion extends and deepens your capacity for caring beyond the defining boundaries of your personal and group identities: "Compassion arises as our response to suffering, period; whose suffering it is should not matter" (Jinpa, 2015, p. 232). Recognizing the universality of suffering (Bridges & Glassman, 2012), you take "it all in. You let the pain of the world touch your heart and you turn it into compassion" (Chödrön, 2016, p. 114). Jinpa (2015) noted that "in Buddhism, one epithet for the Buddha means 'a loving friend even to a stranger', because his compassion is not contingent on any prior history of personal relationship" (pp. 143–144). This puts into context "the Dalai Lama . . . say[ing], 'I have never met anyone who is a stranger'" (Jinpa, 2015, p. 58).

Second, whereas a sympathetic response to another's pain is often perfunctory (a text, a quick call, a tasteful card, a social media post), a compassionate response is more commonly multifaceted and sustained. Compassion involves bearing witness to suffering (Bridges & Glassman, 2012)—staying present for and engaging with it (Davidson & Harrington, 2002, p. 225)—as well as the desire (R. D. Siegel & Germer, 2012, p. 12) and the motivation (Gilbert & Choden, 2014, p. 95; McCall et al., 2014, p. 1) to alleviate it. And compassion tilts toward agency: "Compassion is the triad of *noticing another's suffering, resonating with their suffering in some way*, and then *acting* on [their] behalf" (R. Epstein, 2017, p. 129). According to research by Ervin Staub and his colleagues (as cited in Davidson & Harrington, 2002, p. 226), it is more likely for compassionate desire to become compassionate action when, in addition to being responsive to another's pain, you feel responsible for their welfare.

Compassion in the Buddhist tradition is undergirded by the existential assumption that there is no essential difference between you and anyone else. Makransky (2012) considers it "a cognitive error to think of other beings as intrinsically 'other'" (p. 71). The Tibetan Buddhist teacher Dzigar Kongtrul Rinpoche offered an explanation:

> In Tibetan, we say that all beings with a mind are *drowa semchen*, which means "moving beings." . . . We are all moving, unceasingly, toward what we think will bring us happiness, and away from what we think will make us suffer. No matter how different we look or act, no matter how intelligent or stupid we are, all of us are moving beings. This impulse to move is the very core of our being. . . . Therefore, in our very essence, we are all identical. (Kongtrul, 2016, p. 32, italic in original)

Such equality strips us "of all the categories and labels that we have constructed about ourselves to individuate us from others" (Jinpa, 2015, p. 26).

However, inside your recognition of your and the other's "shared human condition, fragile and imperfect as it is" (Neff, 2012, p. 79), inside the blurred boundary of that mutuality (Jinpa, 2015), compassion, like sympathetic concern, introduces and maintains a subtle but fundamental distinction between you and the person(s) you seek to help. Compassion arises in relation to the other's suffering, not in lockstep with it, so it etches a complementary orientation to—a turning toward—their pain, not a symmetrical entanglement with it (cf. Seikkula et al., 2018, p. 861; in Chapter 2, this volume, I point out that the relational shape of empathy is similarly complementary). What you experience is not the simple mirroring of sympathetic resonance. You feel moved by their pain, and you feel moved to make a difference. This protects you from getting caught up in and taken down by the other's distress.

I described earlier how Carolyn's initial sympathetic resonance with Graham spun into a suffocating, self-conscious panic when, in the midst of their shared sense of us, she slipped into a vivid imagining of herself and her husband in a future replication of Graham's nightmare—of either Art robbed of her, or Art torn from her. Carolyn's panic subsided when she was able to let go of the future and return to the present—back to the living room with Art and her grieving friend. Refocusing on Graham, Carolyn found it possible to once again be there for him, to embrace and tolerate the suffering resonating in the room and registering in her body. But her reengagement raises an important question for all of us. Even if we are able to avoid self-conscious distress altogether, keeping any pain we're witnessing from becoming perilously personal, how sustainable is it to make ourselves emotionally available to clients and patients in pain?

It is well established that there can be a cost to caring (Figley, 2012, pp. 267–269). When you're face to face with others' suffering, particularly for extended periods, the exposure can take a toll, giving rise to caregiver-specific varieties of burnout (Freudenberger, 1974; Kahill, 1988): vicarious trauma (McCann & Pearlman, 1990; Pearlman & Saakvitne, 1995) or compassion fatigue (Figley, 1995; Joinson, 1992). Zaki (2019) referred to compassion fatigue as a "repetitive strain injury" (p. 96), an occupational hazard for "humanity's first responders" (p. 97).

According to Delgado et al. (2023), the culture of health care takes for granted that "physical and emotional exhaustion" is just "part of the job" (p. 460). The prevailing belief is that "compassion requires a willingness on the part of health care providers to be vulnerable, to not only 'feel with' their patient, but also 'suffer with' them, being professionally and personally impacted in the process" (Soto-Rubio & Sinclair, 2018, p. 1431). This helps explain why vicarious trauma among intensive-care professionals, for example, is so high: One in three suffers burnout, and secondary trauma stress (Figley, 2012) afflicts nurses in neonatal intensive care settings almost twice as often as nurses in other settings (Zaki, 2019, p. 103).

It is common for caregivers to attempt to protect themselves from compassion fatigue by suppressing emotions or attempting to gain control over them (Gleichgerrcht & Decety, 2012, p. 252). Zaki (2019) referenced an expert on medical empathy who encourages "caring professionals to adopt what he calls 'detached concern'—a Vulcan sort of goodwill" (p. 102). This term—*detached concern*—goes way back. Renée Fox coined it in 1959 to characterize how physicians must "be sufficiently detached or objective toward the patient to exercise sound medical judgment and maintain . . . equanimity," all the while staying "sufficiently concerned about the welfare of the patient to . . . [provide] compassionate care" (as cited in Cadge & Hammonds, 2012, p. 267). And 70 years before that, in an 1889 address at the University of Pennsylvania, the Canadian "father" of modern North American medicine, Sir William Osler (1904), offered a similar recommendation. He believed physicians, without "hardening the human heart" (p. 5), should have their "nerves well in hand" and their "medullary centres under the highest control" (p. 4) so they could avoid expressing any sign of anxiety or fear. He urged them to strive for "imperturbability" so that "no eventuality [could] disturb [their] mental equilibrium" (Osler, 1904, p. 5) and to "exercise equanimity" "to bear with composure the misfortunes" of their patients (p. 8).

The trouble is, whereas overriding your emotional reactions to patients' and clients' distress may help you cope with their suffering in the short term, reaching for this as a go-to strategy can prove exhausting and alienating (B. B. Davis, 2021, pp. 4–6). It fails to protect against burnout (Halpern, 2001, pp. 15–16) and renders you less effective in your job and less able to handle your frustration (Zaki, 2019, p. 112).

If feeling and suffering with our clients (Soto-Rubio & Sinclair, 2018) threatens our emotional well-being, and, concomitantly, if seeking Osler-style equanimity through emotional detachment carries its own set of comparable risks, then we appear to be caught between a rock and a hard place—between an open heart and a hardened face. Fortunately, there is a third alternative, one that, influenced by Buddhist thought and practices, clearly distinguishes compassion as a commitment to equanimously engaging with and proactively responding to suffering. Buddhist equanimity is achieved "not by detachment due to distancing . . . , nor a desensitized neutrality of feeling" (Olendzki, 2005, p. 296) but by "being present with pleasure without attachment and . . . being present with pain without resistance" (Olendzki, 2010, p. 7). From a Buddhist perspective, the primary way of developing and refining a capacity for equanimous compassion is through meditation (Briere, 2012, p. 274). Chödrön (2016) made clear that "compassionate action is a practice" (p. 103), a practice that, according to R. Epstein (2017), manifests "in surprising and unpredictable ways—through words, small gestures, advocacy, even silence" (p. 129).

Understanding compassion as a learnable skill, Klimecki and Singer (2012) concluded that "the term *compassion fatigue* . . . [is] slightly misleading, since it suggests that caregivers are tired of feeling too much compassion" (p. 378). On the contrary, they said, "the feeling of compassion," (Klimecki & Singer, 2012, p. 378) if it is properly understood and implemented, "should actually protect against burnout" (p. 378). It turns out that the risk to well-being, the risk of burnout, comes not from compassion and not from empathy (Cairns et al., 2024) but, rather, from unmediated empathy-inflected sympathy (Chen et al., 2024)—from what might best be called *resonance fatigue*.

According to Kanske et al. (2015, p. 6), compassion and empathy-inflected sympathy (what they refer to as empathy) rely on different neural networks, a finding that emerged from a series of experiments conducted by Singer and Bolz (2013). It is possible to shift from sympathetic resonance to compassion (Preckel et al., 2018, p. 4), but in the words of the Tibetan Buddhist monk and compassion researcher Matthieu Ricard, empathy-inflected sympathy (what he calls empathy) and the pain that accompanies it "is not a precondition for the arising of compassion" (as cited in Feldman & Kuyken, 2011, p. 118). Batson (2009) similarly pointed out that while sympathetic resonance may serve as a stepping stone to sympathetic concern, it is neither a necessary nor a sufficient precondition. It is possible to feel bad for someone you identify as a friend without necessarily needing to feel as they feel (Batson, 2009, p. 10). As another Tibetan Buddhist monk, quoted by Houshmand et al. (2002), put it, compassion is

> a state "beyond sadness," in which the heart is filled with a desire to help those suffering. In compassion, the sight or contemplation of suffering moves one to action. Sadness, which is passive in comparison, might act as a catalyst or trigger for compassion, but it is a separate and different quality of mind, and the two are not experienced simultaneously but sequentially. Sadness is not a necessary or essential component of compassion; compassion could be experienced with equanimity instead of sadness. (p. 15)

Such equanimity "includes a positive emotional state involving feelings of unconditional caring, kindness, and warmth that are directed to others" (Briere, 2012, p. 267).

Unlike Osler's (1904) self-control approach to achieving dispassionate equanimity, Buddhists "emphasize accepting rather than extirpating emotional reactions" (Halpern, 2001, p. 34, Footnote 1). Instead of striving to keep the other's suffering at bay and your own under wraps, you connect with it, for example, through *tonglen*, a meditation practice and orientation to others that awakens compassionate concern and care (Chödrön, 2016, p. 122). *Tonglen* is a Tibetan word that means giving and taking or sending and receiving. It refers, most generally, to any exchange of self and other (Kongtrul, 2016, pp. 1–2). There are different ways of practicing tonglen meditation, but all involve undertaking some kind of imagined exchange coordinated with the timing of the breath. As you breathe in, you visualize taking in the suffering of one or more others, and as you breathe out, you send them relief (Chödrön, 2016, p. 56) and/or your happiness (Kongtrul, 2016, p. 40).

The psychologist Chris Germer (2012) offered an adaptation of tonglen that involves inhaling "compassion *with* the pain—the medicine along with the toxin" and exhaling "kindness, warmth, and goodwill, effectively reversing our instinctive, and ultimately ruinous, tendency to battle emotional discomfort" (p. 108). As Fischer (2013) put it, the practice of sending and receiving "trains your heart to do what it usually does not want to do: to go toward, rather than away from, what's painful and difficult" (p. 34). It also helps you "to realize that your own suffering and the suffering of others are not different" (Fischer, 2013, p. 34).

Tania Singer (Klimecki et al., 2013) first recognized the different neural signatures of empathy-inflected sympathetic resonance (what she calls empathy) and compassion when she asked Matthieu Ricard to bring his, at that time, 40 years of experience as a monk into her lab. Placing him in a functional MRI (fMRI) machine, she and her colleagues were able to track his brain activity while he meditated. First, for almost an hour, he vividly visualized graphic details of the predicament and suffering of orphaned Romanian children he had seen the night before in a moving television documentary. He later described how intolerable and draining it was to focus on and resonate with their pain for such an extended time: "I felt emotionally exhausted, very similar to being burned out" (Klimecki et al., 2013, p. 471). The researchers were able to see the neural evidence of his distress in the activation of his sympathetic-resonance-for-pain network (what they designated as the "empathy-for-pain network"). Still in the fMRI machine, he then "completely altered [his] mental landscape" (Klimecki et al., 2013, p. 472) by shifting into compassion meditation. Although he continued to envision the children's suffering as vividly as he had previously, the distance between him and the imagined children "completely disappeared" (p. 472). Instead of distress, he felt a "natural and boundless love" for them, along with the "courage to approach and console them" (p. 472). At the neural level, Ricard's compassion meditation activated brain areas that "together form a network related to positive emotions, affiliation and love, and reward" (Klimecki et al., 2013, p. 482).

Tonglen engages the body and imagination in a process of acceptance and proactive transmutation. Breathing in suffering, from both inside and outside your sense of self, you imagine your body transforming it into "lightness, ease, [and] peacefulness" (Fischer, 2013, p. 35), which you then breathe out as relief. Whether undertaken formally as a meditation practice or informally throughout the day, it infuses compassion with agency, the results of which the Zen teacher Norman Fischer (2013) described this way:

> It is enormously helpful to me to no longer feel powerless or at a loss during these difficult times and instead to have a practice that keeps the person constantly on my mind in a way that helps me to feel connected to his or her suffering without feeling enmeshed or capsized by it. (p. 39)

The sympathy you feel for another's plight is an automatic resonance of shared feeling, a boundary-dissolving entrainment that establishes a sense of us. But if it is too intense or sustained too long, it can leave you feeling mired and helpless, needing to pull back or armor up. With compassion, you direct that shared feeling—or a more generalized recognition of universal suffering—into an acknowledgment of shared humanity and a determination to make a difference. This makes it possible to stay present and engaged, if only by imagining your body's receiving and embracing the other's pain, transmuting it, and sending back relief. Like compassion, empathy involves bearing witness, but it channels your resonance with and/or caring for the other into curiosity about them.

A caveat: Some authors (e.g., Bloom, 2016; Fischer, 2013; Gilbert & Choden, 2014) have noted that it is possible to express empathic curiosity about another person without feeling concerned for their well-being. As Kohut (1982) put it, empathy can be pursued "in the service of compassion or hostility. . . . Empathy is never by itself supportive or therapeutic" (p. 397). Thus, in a worst-case scenario, you could empathically delve into another's experience with the nefarious goal of determining how best to torture them (Bloom, 2016, p. 37; Feldman & Kuyken, 2011, p. 117; Fischer, 2013, p. 11; Maibom, 2022, pp. 241–242). Every benevolent human capacity is shadowed by a heartless imposter. As I mentioned earlier, when you drain sympathy of its humanity, you end up with pity. Drain empathy, and you're left with voyeuristic snooping or, worse, what is sometimes called *dark empathy* (Duradoni et al., 2023).

The next chapter delves into the full-hearted version of empathy—a form, as Halpern (2012) said, of *"engaged curiosity"* (p. 237). Your empathic desire to know, oriented by a vision to connect and to help, reaches across the self–other divide to develop an embodied sense and insider appreciation of your client's unique ways of acting, feeling, thinking, choosing, and relating.

2 DEVELOPING EMPATHIC CURIOSITY

One day, I was driving my little boy to school, and I saw this quote by Walt Whitman. It was painted on the wall there. It said, "Be curious, not judgmental."[1] I like that.

—Ted Lasso, in *Ted Lasso* (Bowen & Lowney, 2020)

Or do you wanna be somebody who extends a little empathy to somebody else and, in the process, maybe learn something? Curiosity is the thing that protects you. Curiosity is the thing: It's curative, curiosity.

—Lisa Feldman Barrett, in *Lex Fridman Podcast* (Fridman, 2020)

Just as compassion's commitment is to helping, empathy's is to understanding. Unlike sympathy, empathy doesn't just come to you instantly or spontaneously (Shlien, 1997, p. 73), conjured up by mirror neurons, physical proximity,

---

[1] The codirector of the Walt Whitman Archive, Ed Folsom, has clarified that Whitman never actually said or wrote this (Evon, 2021).

https://doi.org/10.1037/0000472-003
Empathic Engagement in Clinical Practice, by D. Flemons
Copyright © 2026 by the American Psychological Association. All rights reserved.

and/or a caring connection to someone you value. You must, with "mental flexibility," seek out empathic understanding in what is inherently "an effortful and controlled process" (Decety & Jackson, 2004, p. 84). Sympathetic resonance forges an automatic bridge across a self–other difference between like-minded or otherwise similar individuals. It provides a body-based grasp of what someone in the same affective zip code is feeling. But, in keeping with compassion, empathy is capable of taking you further afield, capable of forging a connection not only with something or someone familiar but also different or other, even alien.

Fear, uncertainty, or disgust can prompt you to stay safe by arming up against and backing away from anything or anyone too different, too strange. Curiosity, in contrast, inclines you forward, even into unfamiliar and uncertain territory: "When we're less anxious, defensive, and rigid, curiosity flourishes. Recent research suggests that it also works the other way; the more curious you are, the less anxious, defensive, and rigid you'll be when under psychological stress" (R. Epstein, 2017, p. 47). Empathic curiosity makes it possible for you to wonder, as Einstein did, what you'd observe if you could catch up with and ride alongside a beam of light (Isaacson, 2015) or to imagine what it might be like to be, say, a bat (Nagel, 1974), a wizard (Rowling, 1998), a sparrow (Keats, as cited in Colvin, 1891/2011, p. 48), or an insect (Kafka, 1915/1995).

If, like Carl Rogers (1952), your "major aim is to understand" the other (p. 343), you must bring a heightened attention to your engagement, as well as self-awareness and a commitment to exploration (R. Epstein, 2017, p. 41). Curiosity provides the oomph and direction for your focused attention, but what you come to understand and the nature of your experience along the way will be shaped by the vantage from which you undertake your exploration, what sort of information you seek, and how you venture forth—that is, how you go about gathering information about the other.

Some authors look askance at empathy as a method for knowing others, considering its inherent subjectivity as an inevitable source of bias. Better to aim, so the argument goes, for the kind of rational analysis made possible by viewing, knowing, and making decisions about others from an outside, objective perspective (cf. Bloom, 2016). Objectivity is an ideal that requires you to adopt a perspective that is seemingly located nowhere in particular (Maibom, 2022, p. 33).

Your imagination, integral to all efforts to understand (Flaskas, 2009, p. 151), is always in play, so it is certainly possible to imagine adopting a perspective-free vantage from which to explore clients' experiences. Such is the case for some classical Freudian analysts who, protective of what they perceive to be the scientific status of psychoanalysis, limit their use of empathy as a primary way of knowing (Bohart & Greenberg, 1997a, p. 9; Harari, 1996, p. 56). But as the literary theorist Stanley Fish argued, point of viewlessness doesn't exist (Mina, 2023). The "human point of view is always a view *from somewhere*" (Maibom, 2022, p. 57, italic in original), which can always be nuanced and contextualized by juxtaposing it with any number of other situated perspectives.

Empathy's solution to observer bias is not for you to explore the other's experience from some imagined "neutral" or "objective" nonposition separate from them. With an unapologetic nod to engaged subjectivity (or, as Maibom, 2022, would say, intersubjectivity), empathy offers you a means of exploring a client's experience by establishing and intensifying a connection with and refining your curiosity about them. Carl Rogers (1980) described empathy as a process of entering, making yourself at home, and living temporarily in another's "private perceptual world" (p. 142). His goal was to perceive the emotions and meanings of the client's "internal frame of reference" (p. 140).

Such an approach is possible not only when meeting with an individual client but also when meeting with a family or group. Postmodern family therapists, for example, avoid bias by intentionally adopting multiple perspectives. During therapy sessions, they are able to avoid siding with any one member of a family against other members by empathically listening to and joining with each of them individually. In so doing, they trade out objectivity and detached neutrality for engaged *multipartiality* (e.g., H. Anderson, 1997; H. Anderson & Goolishian, 1988; Hoffman, 1993; Sutherland, 2005). They strive to be on *everyone's* side. I say more about this in Chapter 5.

Theorists vary in how they make sense of the connection, what they seek to understand, how it can best be fashioned, and what can be learned. For Zahavi and Overgaard (2012), empathic curiosity is best directed toward understanding the other's psychological life (p. 7), which, for Maibom (2022), includes homing in on their reasons for thinking, acting (p. 152), and reacting (p. 168) as they do. Adopting an empathic perspective allows you to get a handle on the other's "character, emotions, moods, dispositional tendencies, and life experiences" (Coplan, 2011b, p. 54). Faith T. Fitzgerald (1999) expanded the scope of her empathic curiosity to include an appreciation of the client's context—their "characters, cultures, spiritual and physical responses, hopes, past, and social surrounds" (p. 71). Halpern (2001) sought "an experiential understanding" of the client's "distinct emotional perspective" (p. 68), probing what their emotional response to their circumstances "*is about*" (2012, p. 232). She wants to know how the experience feels.

Empathy-derived understanding reflects the Greek root of the word *know*: *gnōsis*. Plato used this term to refer specifically to sensory-derived knowledge (J. Smeal, personal communication, April 29, 2008): With empathic knowing, you strive to make sense of the other. The understanding you derive and distill is not objective but embodied, not rational but relational. Empathy allows you to get a feel for the interpersonal and intrapersonal relationships interweaving the client's world.

Feeling is a key factor in the world of empathy. After all, grasping how the other feels is critical to your understanding of the heart and encompassment of their psychological life—the reasons for their choices, their orientation to their history, their aspirations, their relationships and culture, as well as how they "think about and react to their . . . emotions" (Willroth et al., 2023, p. 1886, italic in original). But, also, how *you* feel is, or at least can be, pivotal. "Attention without feeling," wrote the poet Mary Oliver, "is only a report" (Popova, 2015).

Theorists and researchers commonly distinguish affective or emotional empathy from cognitive empathy. In broad brushstrokes, the distinction highlights contrasting approaches to data gathering, to different ways of undertaking the task of getting to know someone. With *affective* empathy, your nuanced grasp and appreciation of the other's world is enriched by empathically "feeling your way into" it. You bring your full-bodied engagement into the therapeutic relationship. With *cognitive* empathy—etymology of the word *empathy* be damned[2]—you *think* your way in. You employ reason, prior knowledge of the person, and/or a general grasp of human motivation and beliefs to figure out what they are probably going through and how they're likely responding to it.

Because the distinction between affective and cognitive empathy is so prevalent in the field, particularly in the research literature, it is worthwhile to take a quick look at both terms. I recognize that, as a clinician, you are primarily focused on using whatever information is available—sourced from both your mind and body—to transport your curiosity and imagination from outside to inside the client's world. But let's cleave them (apart) for a moment in preparation for then cleaving them (together).

---

[2]As I explained in Chapter 1, *empathy* derives from the Greek *en*, meaning "in," and *pathos*, meaning "to suffer" or "to feel." It literally, or at least etymologically, means "to feel into."

AFFECTIVE EMPATHY

Stotland (1969) viewed empathy entirely through an affective lens, defining it as "an observer's reacting emotionally because he perceives that another is experiencing or is about to experience an emotion" (p. 272; see also M. H. Davis, 2017). Although the term *affective empathy* is sometimes used to refer to sympathetic concern (Oliver, 2017, p. 177, who calls it empathic concern), it is more typically understood as coming to feel as another person feels through emotion matching or catching (Batson, 2009, pp. 5–6). Many authors (e.g., Coplan, 2011a) pointedly exclude emotional contagion (i.e., the "catching" part of the formulation) as a defining feature of affective empathy, arguing that although empathy involves a sharing of "emotional neural circuits" (J. C. Watson & Greenberg, 2011, p. 133) or "affective neural networks" (de Vignemont & Singer, 2006), the person empathizing, unlike in instances of contagion, recognizes that the other person is the source of the shared feeling (Preckel et al., 2018). The other-focused orientation of affective empathy protects against sympathetic resonance spiraling into self-conscious distress (cf. Zahavi & Overgaard, 2012).

The psychologist Shari Geller once worked with a client struggling in the aftermath of a traumatic car accident. Geller's description of her experience during one of their sessions demonstrates the use of sympathetic resonance as a tool for developing empathic understanding:

> I was seeing my client, L, when I became aware of how an inner emotional sense I was feeling of being overwhelmed was actually my inner resonance of the client's experience. . . . She was describing [some recent, stressful] . . . conversations [she'd had with her boss and her husband] when I became fully present to her experience. I could see her face, sense her holding her breath, her voice was becoming higher in pitch, and I experienced all these without concept or symbol, but more like having them enter me, and I began to feel a sense of what it was like for her. I had this sense in my body of what it is like to feel an overwhelming feeling in one's chest. I became aware of a sense of what it is like to have a panic feeling and did not recognize it as anything familiar in my own experience. I noted that it was an internal resonance to the client's underlying experience. (Geller & Greenberg, 2023, p. 46)

If Geller had lacked the necessary training to employ her sympathetic resonance therapeutically, and if she hadn't developed the capacity to tolerate and make empathic sense of her own resulting heightened affect, she could easily have become overwhelmed by self-conscious personal distress, much the way Carolyn did in Graham's living room (which I described at the beginning of Chapter 1). Instead, appreciating "her own body as a resonator," Geller "receptively opened herself to take in her client's experience."

By remaining "fully grounded and sensing in her own body," she was able "to listen deeply to her own experience," understanding that "her sense of what it was like to feel panic was a present-centered experience of resonance" (Geller & Greenberg, 2023, p. 47).

R. Epstein (2017) described a similar, albeit briefer, encounter between a young physician and his patient that benefited from the doctor's attending to his own affective experience as an attuned instrument of empathy-informed caregiving:

> The resident felt a sinking feeling, a sadness. He wondered whether this feeling was triggered by the patient—whether the patient might be depressed or even suicidal—which then tripped his internal circuit breaker and captured his attention. In fact, the patient *was* depressed. . . . The resident's ability to pick up on this signal was a direct result of his awareness of his own emotions—the heaviness he felt only grew stronger the more he talked with the patient. . . . He used his own emotions to inform his care of the patient. (p. 28)

In Chapter 3, I return to the idea of turning toward your personal affective experience, whether an artifact of sympathetic resonance or the result of your concern for the client (or both), and utilizing it to enhance your empathic connection and understanding.

COGNITIVE EMPATHY

Cognitive empathy theorists and researchers conceive of empathy primarily, and sometimes even solely, as a thinking process or reaction (M. H. Davis et al., 1987), undertaken through perspective-taking or role-playing (Eisenberg et al., 1991). Explanations for how it works draw on two principal theories. The first proposes that when you're cognitively empathizing, you're theoretically teasing out—deducing or making inferences about—the other person's perspective, including their beliefs, intentions, needs, and/or feelings (Preckel et al., 2018; Shamay-Tsoory, 2009). This is conventionally termed the "theory of mind" (ToM) or mindreading explanation (Zahavi & Overgaard, 2012) or, with no apparent self-aware irony, the "theory theory" explanation. Some authors, in line with Dymond (1949) and Borke (1971), go so far as to argue that, in constructing for yourself another's mental state, it is possible to remain completely devoid of feeling (e.g., Currie, 2004, as cited in Feagan, 2011, p. 150, Footnote 2; see also A. Smith, 2006). In other words, you can go ahead and consider the other's affect as relevant to their experience if you want, but your affect isn't necessary for—and can muck up—your experience of scoping out theirs. The idea that this is even possible, that a therapist could empathize with a client without breaking an affective sweat, reflects dueling dualistic assumptions about the separability of emotion and reason and the separability of each person in the interaction as if they were autonomous automatons (cf. O'Hara, 1997, p. 313). More on that a little later.

This affect-free conception of empathy surfaces in medical practice and education, where clinicians and students are advised "to recognize and name another's distress as an emotion without experiencing that state themselves" (R. Epstein, 2017, p. 131; see also Halpern, 2012, p. 230). Shapiro (2012) explained the rationale for "taming" empathy in this way, for keeping it safe and predictable:

> An understanding of empathy that relies solely on cognitive processes seems more controllable, more manageable, more teachable, and more measurable in terms of outcomes. The result has been to promote empathy as a kind of cognitive listening to and apprehension of the patient's concerns while avoiding the perceived "risks" of emotional involvement with the patient. (p. 278)

The second explanation for how cognitive empathy works invokes the notion of *simulation*. This theory proposes that you internally represent the other's mental states by "tracking or matching those states with resonant states" of your own (Shamay-Tsoory, 2009, p. 216). Most theorists agree that cognitive empathy necessitates a combination of ToM theorizing and simulation (Spaulding, 2017). Alvin I. Goldman (2011, p. 38), for example, described what he calls "high-level" simulation, which involves using previously attained information to help you imaginatively reproduce and reexperience in your mind the state of mind of the other.

If simulation involves imagining what you would think, feel, and do if you were to be in the other's shoes (Spaulding, 2017, p. 15), then you can't undertake it without engaging neural networks associated with emotion processing (Shamay-Tsoory, 2009): "Mental imagery not only enables us to see the world of our conspecifics through their eyes or as if in their shoes, but may also result in similar sensations as the other person's" (Decety & Lamm, 2009, p. 201). The simulation explanation of cognitive empathy thus serves as a bridge between cognitive and affective empathy. Shamay-Tsoory (2009) speculated that simulation-based cognitive empathy and affective empathy come online when you and the other share experiences and an emotional relationship. When you and the other are more emotionally and experientially distant, ToM-based cognitive empathy would be more likely to kick in (pp. 227–228).

Clearly, some cognitive-empathy theorists consider the therapist's affect to be a not-always-necessary but sometimes-maybe-helpful contribution to empathically understanding the client. This sounds reasonable enough.

The trouble is that the cleaving of empathy into distinct cognitive and affective domains reflects a long-held, problematic assumption about the relationship between mind and body and, downstream from that, the relationship between cognition and emotion or between rationality and irrationality. Let's dig into that a little, if only so that when we emerge from the discussion, you can wrap both your head and your arms around an appreciation of empathy as a thoroughly mind–body enterprise.

COGNITION AND AFFECT

We have invented or borrowed from Descartes an idea about a separation between something which is of one nature, mind, and something of another nature, body. From there on, [we] cannot make any sense of anything.
—Gregory Bateson, in Robert W. Rieber's *The Individual, Communication, and Society* (1989, p. 328)

René Descartes (1641/1911), the 17th-century philosopher and mathematician, famously argued that mind is fundamentally different from and independent of the body, writing in his "Meditation VI,"

> Because . . . I have a clear and distinct idea of myself . . . as . . . a thinking and unextended thing, and . . . I possess a distinct idea of body, inasmuch as it is only an extended and unthinking thing, it is certain that this I . . . is entirely and absolutely distinct from my body, and can exist without it. (p. 28)

Bloom (2016) considered the dichotomy between reason and emotion an inherent opposition at the core of human nature. It is, he said, the oldest and most resilient of all psychological theories. In fact, it predates Descartes by a couple of thousand years. According to Barrett (2017a, Introduction, para. 10), Descartes was only echoing what Plato, Hippocrates, and Aristotle had much earlier proposed. Regardless of when it was first articulated or later elaborated, this dualistic artifact of Greek and proto-Enlightenment thought doesn't hold up in the face of current neurological evidence. Given the structure of the brain, it is clear that "rationality and emotion are not at war" (Barrett, 2020, p. 16). According to Duncan and Barrett (2007), "there is no such thing as a 'non-affective thought'" (pp. 1–2). And affect, a core contributor to sensory experience, consciousness, language, and memory, is, itself, "a form of cognition" (Duncan & Barrett, 2007, p. 12).

We commonly assume that what you feel is influenced by your perceptions of the outside world; however, Barrett (2017a) pointed out that this characterization is mostly backward. What you feel alters what you perceive and think, and it alters how you decide and act: "Affect is in the driver's seat and rationality is a passenger" (p. 79). This is because "the human brain is anatomically structured so that no decision or action can be free of interoception and affect, no matter what fiction people tell themselves about how rational they are" (pp. 81–82).

If every cognition has an affective spin and every affect is cognitively spun, the dualistic split between cognitive and affective empathy risks being misconceived as a black-and-white, absolute division. The two are mutually defining complements, not independent opposites. To better convey that the distinction is more conceptual invention than biological truth, we would be better off referring to cognitive empathy as *affect-attenuated* empathy and affective empathy as *cognition-attenuated* empathy. We'd also be wise to take a closer look at what emotions are and how they work.

First, though, a suggestion: Before reading on, you might want to grab a coffee and buckle up—what follows is a bit of a wild ride. And prepare yourself for when you disembark: You'll begin to see empathy in a whole new light, with implications that will reverberate through the rest of the book.

THE THEORY OF CONSTRUCTED EMOTION

Feeling something [is] . . . never simply a state of submission but always, also, a process of construction.

—Leslie Jamison, *The Empathy Exams* (2014)

Much of the research on empathy is informed not only by a presumed ontological separation between reason and affect but also by what Barrett (2017a) called the "classical model of emotion," an essentialist characterization that conceives of emotions as inherited, preestablished neural signatures that are triggered by outside circumstances, are experienced automatically in the body, and are physically manifested and thus observable in characteristic and definable facial expressions. The classical model, which has been thoroughly and extensively researched (e.g., Ekman, 2021), takes for granted that emotions are universally consistent across individuals and cultures (Gündem et al., 2022). Coplan (2011a) exemplified the essentialist position in her assertion that fundamentally distinct "basic emotions"—such as, for example, fear, anger, sadness, joy, and disgust—are cross-culturally experienced. Ekman and Cordaro (2011) mostly concurred but substituted happiness for joy and added contempt to this list.

However, according to Barrett (2017a), brain research has firmly established that the classical model is incorrect. Emotions do not have distinct essences in the form of dedicated neural circuits, responsible genes, or innate "programs" (p. 157). Rather, emotions, like perceptions, are constructed. According to Barrett's (2017a) theory of constructed emotion, "an emotion is your brain's creation of what your bodily sensations mean, in relation to what is going on around you in the world" (p. 30).

Your brain is continually making internal adjustments to systems, organs, tissues, and processes throughout your body, and as it does this, it predicts the sensory consequences of these changes. Meanwhile, it is receiving moment-by-moment updates on the internal functioning of the body, and it uses this information to confirm or correct its predictions and to tweak, if necessary, the change signals it is sending back out (Barrett, 2017a, 2017b; Barrett & Quigley, 2021). This process of predicting, sensing, comparing, and adjusting involves an integration of *allostasis* (the efficient prediction and regulation of metabolism and energy) and *interoception* (sensations that arise from ongoing allostatic tinkering, many of which you're not consciously aware; Barrett et al., 2016). The brain translates interoception signals into consciously available internal feeling or affect, which becomes a key ingredient in the construction of emotion (Barrett, 2017a, p. 56).

You notice and register simple affect as a point along two intersecting continuums—*valence* (how pleasant or unpleasant you feel) and degree of *arousal* or *activation* (how calm or jazzed or agitated you feel). Pleasant valence and high activation is experienced as elation, pleasant valence and mid-activation as feeling pleased or gratified, pleasant valence and low activation as calmness or serenity, unpleasant valence and low activation as lethargy or depression, unpleasant valence and mid-activation as misery, and unpleasant valence and high activation as upset or distress (see Barrett, 2017a, p. 74).[3] As with everyone else in your and others' culture, basic feelings of pleasure and displeasure continually and pervasively inform your everyday experience (Barrett, 2017a, p. 56), inclining you in a knee-jerk way toward happiness and away from suffering (Kongtrul, 2016, pp. 31–32).

In your everyday life, you are buffeted about in this way, just like everyone else; however, when you're engaging with others as a therapist, a health care professional, or anyone else offering compassionate care, a zap of unpleasant feeling can become a valuable source of information to be tolerated and

---

[3] See Barrett and Russell (1998) for an earlier, somewhat different iteration of this model; see Kuppens et al. (2013) for research on differences in how the two properties interrelate, depending on both the individual and the circumstances.

investigated. Ron Epstein (2017), a family physician, explained how, in the midst of, or even after, examining a patient, his clinical acumen is informed by his affect:

> Every once in a while . . . [a patient] with symptoms similar to those of a virus has something more serious. In those situations, something doesn't feel quite right to me. I feel a sense of unease. My brain is on high alert, yet the accompanying feelings are visceral and hard to describe—I just don't feel comfortable inside. . . . It would be so easy to ignore the feeling and move along to the next task. But I'm curious when a patient "looks sick." . . . I am attuned in a way that invites further exploration, often before I can characterize why. (pp. 40–41)

But whereas simple affect is universal, emotions are not. As Mesquita (2022) explained,

> Emotions such as *anger, shame, love,* or *happiness* do not have universal signatures. Instead, the experience and expression, the associated physiological and neural response patterns, and the moral connotations and social consequences are different across instances, individuals, interactions, relationships, and of course, cultures. (p. xi, italic in original)

Contrary to both the classical model and what intuitively feels true, an emotion is not a thing, not a prefab, stored expression waiting in the wings to be activated when circumstances warrant or trigger it. Rather, it is a constructed "category of instances, and any emotion category has tremendous variety" (Barrett, 2017a, p. 16). On "different occasions, in different contexts, . . . within the same individual and across different individuals, the same emotion category involves different bodily responses" (Barrett, 2017a, p. 15), including facial expressions. An emotion like fear "does not have a single expression but a *diverse population of facial movements* that vary from one situation to the next" (Barrett, 2017a, p. 10, italic in original). And the same is true of happiness, sadness, anger, and so on.

When an emotional expression arises in you, unbidden, it is spontaneously constructed and uniquely expressed, and it shapes—perhaps even defines—how you're understanding whatever you're currently encountering. It orients you. But the occurrence and perspective-shaping nature of the emotion is itself also an expression of how you're construing this experience in relation to past, analogous situations. Feeling and concept—sense and sensemaking—entangle. As William Blake (ca. 1803) articulated in his poem "The Grey Monk," "A tear is an intellectual thing" (p. 13). Experiencing an emotion involves giving lightning-fast, present-moment meaning to your interoceptive sensations and affect, influenced by the context, by a lifetime of experience, and courtesy of your culture and language, by names and concepts (emotion categories) baked into your sensibility. This is true of everyone—you, your colleagues, and your clients.

Barrett's theory of constructed emotion marks a paradigm shift (Kuhn, 2012), not only in understanding emotion but also in the conception and practice of empathy. As you sit across from a client, you can no longer assume that your goal is to read facial expressions, voice quality, posture, gestures, and so on as outer signs of a discrete, universally felt inner emotion. The challenge to this assumption implicates the whole notion of empathic accuracy (more on that in just a moment); however, the theory also opens the door to a reconception of what an empathic statement is. If there is no stand-alone source emotion inside the client for you to tap into, identify, and reflect back, what's going on during empathic conversations? How do we make sense of and engage in empathic listening? As I explain in Chapter 5, if emotions are constructed, our listening to our clients isn't reflective; it's *refractive*. You and the client working together to put their experience into words coconstruct a felt meaning that combines discovery and invention. The therapeutic implications of this recognition (which I also discuss in Chapter 5) are significant and far-reaching.

EMPATHIC ACCURACY

All empathic responses are inherently tentative, implying the therapist's asking the client, "Is this accurate?"
—Jerold D. Bozarth, Empathy From the Framework of Client-Centered Theory and the Rogerian Hypothesis (1997, p. 93)

The theory of constructed emotion shakes the ground under the research on *accurate empathy* (Rogers, 1957) or *empathic accuracy* (Ickes, 1997; Ickes et al., 1990), a measure of the ability to infer another's thoughts and feelings. Research suggests that with a stranger, empathic inference will be accurate about 20% of the time; with a close friend, your accuracy could rise to 30%; and if you attempt it with your life partner, you'll max out at 35% (Ta & Ickes, 2017, p. 355). Why so low? Ickes (2011) speculated that evolution has played a role in "calibrat[ing the] ceiling" of empathic accuracy (p. 201). If our forebears' accuracy had been too high, he suggested, they would have been inclined to give too much weight to others' interests, jeopardizing their own interests and, thus, their survival.

A simpler explanation that avoids the teleological complexities of evolutionary-psychology speculations can be derived from the theory of constructed emotion. You may sympathetically resonate with another's affect—with the valence and degree of activation characterizing their feeling;

however, such resonance doesn't give you privileged access to the contextualizing, categorizing, and sensemaking involved in their emotional experience. Contrary to what Zaki et al. (2008) asserted, you can't "directly experience" (p. 399) their emotions.

> You *need* an emotion concept in order to experience or perceive the associated emotion. It's a requirement. Without a concept for "Fear," you cannot experience fear. Without a concept for "Sadness," you cannot perceive sadness in another person. . . . Your brain must be able to make that concept and predict with it. Otherwise, you will be experientially blind to that emotion. (Barrett, 2017a, p. 141, italic in original)

No emotion concept has a consistent, predetermined neural pattern or a fixed visual or audible representation, so neither the facial expressions and gestures you see nor the paralinguistic cues you hear offer you definitive, identifiable indicators of some standard-issue emotion that the other is currently experiencing. Empathy researchers have run up against this disconnect between the thoughts and emotions that people are feeling and what shows up on their faces and in their gestures:

> Nonverbal expressions of intentions, beliefs, and emotions often fail to match the states [people] . . . are actually experiencing. . . . Even while experiencing powerful emotions, [people] . . . often produce subtle cues that leave perceivers puzzling over what those targets are feeling. (Zaki & Ochsner, 2011, pp. 162–163)

As the person in front of you spontaneously constructs the instance of emotion they're feeling, you spontaneously construct your perception of it. It is thus an error to "speak of perceiving someone's emotion 'accurately'. Instances of emotion have no objective fingerprints in the face, body, and brain, so 'accuracy' has no scientific meaning. . . . Perceptions exist within the perceiver" (Barrett, 2017a, p. 39).

Zaki et al. (2008, p. 399) expressed surprise that researchers have not yet been able to convincingly demonstrate a tangible relationship between affective (cognition-attenuated) empathy, which he defines as feeling with the other, and cognitive (affect-attenuated) empathy, the ability to infer the thoughts and emotions of another person accurately. But if you recognize that emotions aren't pressed and hanging on a rack in our brains, ready to be slipped into and displayed for all to see, then the lack of association between resonance and inference becomes understandable. Sympathetic attunement with a client establishes a sensory connection with them, but this, in itself, doesn't communicate the details, the felt meaning (Rogers, 1980) of their emotion. Because resonance alone doesn't convey the emotion concept the client is constructing out of the valance and activation level of the affect (cf. Halpern, 2001, p. 79), you can only speculate how they're emotionally making sense of their sensory experience.

> Perceptions of emotions are guesses, and they're "correct" only when they match the other person's experience; that is, both people agree on which [emotion] concept to apply. Anytime you think you know how someone feels, your confidence has nothing to do with actual knowledge. (Barrett, 2017a, p. 195)

Lewis and Hodges (2012) also acknowledged the limits of perception for getting a handle on another person's emotional experience, suggesting that imagining the other's experience may get you further than simply honing your perceiving (p. 74). But although imaginatively taking the perspective of another person can increase your confidence in the accuracy of your empathic understanding, you should, Barrett suggested, remain wary of your certainty. Eyal et al. (2018) found that while perspective-taking improves your bond with the other person, it can decrease your empathic accuracy. The only thing that can improve accuracy is perspective *getting*, which you acquire through conversation. According to Ta and Ickes (2017), empathic accuracy depends most on what the other says and how they say it; nonverbal cues are least important (pp. 357–358). As Maibom (2022) put it, "Flatfooted though it may seem, asking others what's on their minds is doubtless the gold standard for understanding them" (p. 167).

This book is about *empathic engagement*, about how to develop and refine empathic understanding *in conversation* with others, so of course, I agree that talking is gold, but I'm not sure what's flatfooted about such an acknowledgment. Rogers asserted that empathy is as much a dialogical as a psychological process (Cissna & Anderson, 2002). He realized that empathy requires "frequently checking with the [other] person as to the accuracy" of what you're coming to understand, which allows you to be "guided by the responses you receive" (Rogers, 1980, p. 142).

Because of the range of variability in the constructing and expressing of emotion, both within and across individuals, there is no "emotion circuit" in the brain of your client that can serve as a benchmark against which your "empathic accuracy" can be objectively measured. However, when you offer empathic comments in a therapeutic conversation, your client is perfectly positioned to juxtapose what you say with how they're making sense of what they're thinking and feeling. This allows them to assess—and express—the degree to which your offerings are spot on or off the mark. As Frankel (2017) put it, "The criterion for empathic accuracy/effectiveness lies in the sequence of exchanges not simply the words in isolation" (p. 2130). If you adjust your empathic understanding in response to the client's feedback, your accuracy can improve over the course of the conversation (Ta & Ickes, 2017, p. 357). I return to this issue in Chapter 5.

SPARKING THE EMPATHIC IMAGINATION

Empathy is a kind of imagining.
—Murray Smith, *Empathy, Expansionism, and the Extended Mind* (2011, p. 100)

Capacities to "wonder," to "wait in uncertainties," to imagine into the life of the other, are . . . vital for the creative work of the great writer. They are also vital parts of the capacity for empathy and for therapy.
—Ron Perry, *Empathy—Still at the Heart of Therapy* (1993, p. 69)

The imagination is the single most useful tool humankind possesses. It beats the opposable thumb. . . . The imagination is a fundamental way of thinking, an essential means of becoming and remaining human.
—Ursula K. Le Guin, *The Wave in the Mind* (2004, p. 202)

Empathy is a means of getting a feel for and making sense of another person's experience, choices, actions, anticipations, responses, and reasons within the context of their history, circumstances, and/or relationships. Opinions and theories vary significantly about how empathy is sparked and where it leads you. Zaki (2019) considered sympathetic resonance (what he called "experience sharing") to be empathy's "leading edge" (p. 179). It *can* be, but there is no single, accepted way to spark your empathic engagement with another person (Halpern, 2001, p. 92).

Sitting across from a distraught client, you might immediately sense a sympathetic resonance arising in you, a shared feeling of upset or unease that can serve as a doorway into their world (Hill-hain & Rogers, 1988, p. 69). Alternatively, it might be sympathetic concern—your compassionate caring about their distress (Halpern, 2012, p. 238)—that first grabs you and launches your empathic exploration. And, then again, your initial empathic impulse may be, for whatever reason, an affect-attenuated reaching fueled by a dispassionate interest (cf. Stueber, 2006). Regardless of what serves as the leading edge of your empathic imagination (Margulies, 1989)—shared affect (sympathetic resonance), sympathetic concern, or simply a desire to know—your making sense of the other will be most comprehensive when all three contribute to the process, that is, when your curiosity is compassionate and viscerally informed (cf. Shapiro, 2012). As Greenberg and Elliott (1997) put it,

> A therapist often experiences a complex felt sense, a complex sense of understanding the felt meaning of the situation of the client. What is important is that it is something the therapist feels rather than just understands intellectually. Empathy is . . . [an] experiential process of understanding. (p. 169)

Halpern (2001) noted that "although both empathy and sympathy involve emotional resonance, . . . empathy involves using resonance to attune to another's specific emotional views through imagination" (p. 87). Empathic imagining provides context and specific content for what is felt, whether or not it is triggered by resonance.

Okay, but imagine what, exactly? What's the most efficient and effective way to envision crossing the self–other boundary? Like everything else in the field, opinions vary, but by far, the most accepted method is to imagine beaming yourself, Star Trek style, into the precise circumstances—indeed, into the very shoes—of the other person.

IN-THE-SHOES IMAGINATION

Before you criticize a man, walk a mile in his shoes. That way, if he's upset, he's a mile away and you've got his shoes.
    −Johnny Carson, in *The Tonight Show* (Carson, 1991)

The adage that we should not judge another person until we've walked a mile in their shoes would benefit from more thought.
    −Ellen J. Langer, *The Mindful Body* (2023, p. 64)

Empathy always involves an imaginative foray across a self–other boundary—a conjured excursion to acquire and develop a felt understanding of the other's experience. During an empathic undertaking, you can always draw on various aspects of your self—your personal history, your values, your expert knowledge, your intra- and interpersonal sensitivity—as points of comparison for perceiving and making sense of the other. But it is worthwhile to question when, how, and, indeed, even if it is helpful to explicitly bring this sense of self along for the ride, keeping it forefront in your mind as you explore the other's world.

Many clinicians and authors employ the image of "walking in another's shoes" when conceiving of, researching, and/or practicing empathy (e.g., Decety & Lamm, 2009; Fliess, 1942; Goldie, 2011; Greenberg & Elliott, 1997; Kongtrul, 2016; Lewis & Hodges, 2012; Maibom, 2022; Mina, 2023; Preston et al., 2007; Segal et al., 2017; M. Smith, 2011). Implicit in this cliché is the idea that you come to understand the other by imaginatively parachuting your intact, circumscribed self—complete with your history of being in the world in your embodied way (cf. M. Smith, 2011, p. 105)—into their context, facing their challenges and choices. You "imagine what thoughts, feelings, decisions, and so on *you* would arrive at if you were in the other's circumstances" (Goldie, 2011, p. 302). This generates what is best thought of as *analogy-inflected empathy*—attempting empathic understanding of the client by treating your embodied experience as functionally analogous to theirs.

Maibom (2022) offered a hack to employ if, while engaged in in-the-shoes empathizing, you were to encounter someone to whom you couldn't directly relate. She described the plight of a socially conservative straight man attempting to take the perspective of a gay man by imagining having sex with a male partner. Because the straight man, himself, does not desire men, Maibom opined, he cannot "realign . . . his interests with those of the other person" (Maibom, 2022, p. 133). The hack encourages the straight man to think analogically, to substitute the other's source of arousal with his own: "Instead of imagining having sex with someone he does not sexually desire," Maibom (2022) suggested, "he should imagine having sex with someone he loves" (p. 133).[4] This appeal to comparison accords with Buie's model of "resonant empathy." Buie's idea was to empathically infer an understanding of a patient's personal world by turning inward, searching your memories for "configurations of experience" that might give rise to the sorts of behaviors, communications, and emotions you're observing in the other (Bohart & Greenberg, 1997a, p. 11).

An in-the-shoes style of empathic engagement, outfitted with such analogy-generating strategies for rendering too-different differences more palatable, or at least more imaginable, allows you to keep your sense of self close at hand, filtering the other's circumstances and experiences through your standards of what's normal, acceptable, and/or possible (cf. Langer, 2023, pp. 64–65).

---

[4]Maibom could have more broadly referenced the challenge of in-the-shoes empathizing with anyone whose object of desire or source of pleasure is different from your own.

But in so doing, you risk hollowing out the wholeness of the client's living, breathing personhood, relegating the other to little more than a placeholder or a shell for you to embody (cf. to Arthur Koestler's characterization of empathy as a "projection of part of our own personality into the shell of the other," as cited in Lanzoni, 2018, p. 211).

The limitations of practicing this approach to empathy come into sharp focus if you tag it as a cousin of anthropomorphism. Say you're a naive equestrian struggling to saddle a mare who is agitating against your every move. If you were to attempt a little in-the-(horse)shoes imagining, analogically bringing your values and motivations into your surmising, you might suspect that her lack of cooperation is motivated by jealousy and spite. After all, did she not witness you earlier in the day riding a gelding with whom she shares a paddock? The thing is, horses don't think, feel, or respond in any way resembling this characterization (see Hötzel et al., 2019; Lesté-Lasserre, 2019), so your suspicions would not only be inadequate but also woefully, ridiculously wrong.

Halpern (2012) noted that "it can be tempting for [a] . . . doctor to imagine *herself* in a patient's shoes and think that she knows how the patient feels because of how *she* (the doctor) would feel" (p. 237, italic in original); however, such an act of imagination will fall short of illuminating the lived experience of the other. Coplan (2011b) called this style of engagement *pseudo-empathy* (p. 54). If taken to an extreme, it could devolve into what might best be termed *selfie empathy*—treating the client's world as an exotic locale and backdrop against which you focus and document your self-conscious presence. Although the capacity to distinguish a sense of self in the midst of empathizing is essential for keeping your wits about you (Krol & Bartz, 2022), keeping it front and center can limit your attempts to understand the other, and it can throw your well-being into disarray, as it did my clinical graduate student, Michelle.

One semester, Michelle started working with a socially isolated 17-year-old girl, Chelsea, who had recently suffered three significant losses. An excellent athlete, Chelsea had been the star wing spiker on the varsity volleyball team, but a serious injury had benched her for at least the rest of the season. In addition, her somewhat estranged father had died a few months earlier, and still more recently, her boyfriend had broken up with her. Worried about Chelsea's possible suicidality, Michelle was frightened that her efforts to help could, if bungled, put her client at greater risk. She had reason to be afraid: Michelle was struggling like crazy to connect with Chelsea empathically, but the more she tried, the more shut down Chelsea became. I was concerned about Chelsea but also about Michelle.

I asked Michelle what was going on for her as she sat across from her client. She replied,

> My father is such an important person in my life. I can't imagine what I'd do if I were to lose him now, never mind what effect this would have had if I were still 17. And then, on top of that, if I can't play my most loved sport and my boyfriend dumps me? . . . I see Chelsea in . . . [the therapy room], thinking about all she is facing, and I have tears but no words. I just feel so bad for her.

Choked up by her sympathetic resonance and her feet crammed into Chelsea's shoes, Michelle was using her empathic imagination to conjure an analogy-based parallel universe where she, like her client, was struggling to cope with overwhelming losses that were personal to her. It was peopled with Michelle's loved ones, not Chelsea's. So she was trying to help her client while marinating in a virtual reality where her dad had died, where she had been dumped, where she was incapable of playing a sport crucial to her identity. The virtual reality she conjured for herself felt so tangible and overwhelming that it left her almost speechless. Coupled with that, she was left feeling guilty for having led such a privileged life: "I'm trying to learn, . . . figure out, get information from her, and . . . it's like, you know, I didn't have to deal with . . . [what she's facing], and I just feel really guilty because she did, or she does."

Michelle's experience raises the question of emotional safety in the practice of empathy. I return to this early in the next chapter, where I focus on issues and offer practices related to self-care. But for those discussions to make sense, we first need to look at variations in what happens to the boundary of your self and your concomitant self-awareness, depending on how you undertake the challenge of empathically crossing the self–other border. Rather than attempting an analogical appreciation of the client by beaming your sense of self into their shoes, it is possible (and preferable) to undertake a *metaphoric* understanding by projecting your self-less imagination into their circumstances and embodied experience.

METAPHORIC IMAGINATION

Metaphor is not just pretty poetry, it is not either good or bad logic, but is in fact . . . the main characteristic and organizing glue of [the] . . . world of mental process.

—Gregory Bateson & Mary Catherine Bateson, *Angels Fear* (1987, p. 30)

You can't reverse . . . metaphors. While you can say "He's clean" to mean he has no criminal record, you can't say "He's moral" to mean that he bathed recently. Metaphor is unidirectional.
                                —Benjamin K. Bergen, Metaphors Are in the Mind (2013, p. 219)

In line with Theodor Lipps's defining Einfühlung as a fusion of self and other (see Chapter 1 and Lanzoni, 2018, p. 33), Mahrer (1997) characterized empathy as "a washing away of the self–other distinction" (p. 200; see also Zaki, 2019, p. 179). In stark contrast, Zahavi and Overgaard (2012) asserted that empathy requires a clear conception of the other as separate from you, as not you: "The experience you empathically understand remains that of the other. The focus is on the other, and the distance between self and other is preserved and upheld" (p. 6). Coplan (2011b) likewise underscored the necessity of clear boundaries: Empathy demands, she said, that you "attend to relevant differences between self and other" (pp. 58–59).

So which is it? In empathy, do self and other merge? Or diverge? Is the boundary between self and other dissolved? Or distinguished? The answer is yes—not to either one *or* the other, not to one *then* the other, but to both simultaneously. In empathy, self and other merge *and* diverge; the boundary between them is dissolved *and* distinguished.

There's something oddly paradoxical about this. Lanzoni (2018) alluded to it when explaining that empathy "marks a relation between the self and other that draws a border but also builds a bridge. . . . If at first we might see empathy as a sharing of similarities, empathy also hinges on difference" (pp. 17–18). A historian, Lanzoni (2018), noted that "over the past one hundred years, empathy has conveyed notions of fusion, identity, and similarity as well as projection, separation, and difference. Empathy matches one's experience to something or someone else, but it also marks difference" (p. 278).

A few authors have attempted to rescue empathy from paradox by inserting time or rationality into its formulation. For example, in her depiction of the imagination required of therapists when they are forging an empathic connection, Flaskas (2009) described the necessity of "a back-and-forth movement between the fantasy of sameness and the fantasy of difference" (p. 153). The therapist doesn't imagine being simultaneously identical to and different from the client and doesn't imagine the impossibility of being one with the client while remaining separate from the client. Instead, the therapist imagines alternating between identity and difference—first the same, then different, then the same, then different. The oscillation renders impossibility possible.

Meissner (2010) staked out comparable territory by trading the paradoxical imagination of identity for the rational imagination of similarity. "My . . . empathic attunement with my patient, involves a . . . complex sense of myself as *like* [emphasis added] but also *unlike* [emphasis added] the other" (Meissner, 2010, p. 429). This conception of empathy nests comfortably inside the logic of *simile*, where similarity and difference go hand in hand; they live side by side. By being like his patient in some ways, he is, of course, unlike the patient in a host of others.

The inherent rationality of simile also informs Maibom's (2022) in-the-shoes empathy hack I mentioned earlier. If Maibom is right that a straight man can only successfully empathize with a gay man's experience of sex if he imagines himself with a lover that he himself desires, then, so too, a gay man wishing to empathize with a straight man would need to imagine sex with a male, not a female, lover. Both men are similar in their capacity for arousal, but because they differ in terms of the gender of the partner to which they're attracted, they each, according to Maibom, must make a mental substitution if they are to appreciate the experience of the other's desire. Clearly, analogy-based imagined switching would be necessary not only in this instance but also in all simile-grounded empathizing, given that we all differ from each other in significant ways. Recognizing the limits of a simile-structured imagining of another person's point of view, Maibom (2022) advised that "it is neither possible, nor desirable, to attempt to imagine being that person in all their distinctiveness" (p. 33). Still, if you remain steadfastly *you* as you imaginatively traipse around in the other's shoes, you may get a handle on what they're facing, but their experience of their circumstances will elude you.

So what would happen if you didn't bother trying to eschew the paradox of empathy? What happens if you don't shuffle back and forth between imagining the client as the same as, and then different from, you? Or if you don't strive to preserve the defining boundaries and guiding principles of your sense of self by making analogy-based adjustments in your imagination of the other? Embracing paradox, rather than trying to avoid it, takes you beyond toe-dipping empathy (cf. Mahrer, 1997, p. 200); it constructs a radical, all-in empathy—empathy not tamed by simile but electrified by metaphor. Drawing on philosopher Ted Cohen's ideas about metaphors of "interpersonal imagining" (2008) and "personal identification" (1999), we could say that empathy can be imagined as a metaphoric identification with the client, in which self isn't *like* the other, self *is* the other. I imagine not that I am in some ways like you (and, therefore, in other ways unlike you) but that I *am* you (e.g., Coplan, 2011b, p. 54; Hojat, 2016, p. vii; Lu, 2021).

Here is where the paradox of empathy most clearly spins into view. When I'm imagining that I am you, "no subject-object separation" exists (Bridges &

Glassman, 2012, p. 146). We are one. Nevertheless, Theodor Lipps and Rollo May's claims notwithstanding (Lanzoni, 2018, p. 205), metaphoric identity does not produce a simple fusion. When I empathically imagine being you, my articulation of this idea necessarily involves delineating the two individual elements—self and other, I and you—composing it. Thus, I can't imagine that you and I are ONE without referencing the *two* of us: "*I AM you.*" In denying the boundary between self and other, empathy as metaphor indirectly but inevitably, simultaneously and paradoxically invokes it. Just as every explicit duality is an implicit unity (Watts, 1975, p. 26), you can't explicitly dismiss difference without implicitly underscoring it (see Flemons, 1991, 2002).

A radical conception of empathy opens up the possibility of your exploring the world of the other without your circumscribed self grabbing the steering wheel or even coming along for the ride. When undertaking simile-and/or analogy-based empathic imagining, you continually harken back to your history, values, antipathies, and proclivities to establish points of comparison for taking the measure of the other's experience. As you're imaginatively slipping into their shoes or, Freaky Friday style, inhabiting their body,[5] you etch your empathic understanding through the ongoing explicit juxtaposition of self and other.

When undertaking metaphor-based empathic imagining, you still retain the capacity to, at any point, redirect your focus back to yourself. As I explained in Chapter 1, self and other are relationally interdependent, so a sense of self is necessarily invoked, if only implicitly, any time you're distinguishing something or someone other. However, knowing you can turn back to yourself for orienting reference doesn't mean you must. It is possible to absorb yourself in the details of the other's experience so that self-conscious awareness and concern become mostly unnecessary and irrelevant. As your imagination of being the other is nuanced and elaborated, the need to harken back to a circumscribed self is enervated. Just slip on your invisibility cloak (Rowling, 1998), and off you go (cf. Rogers [1980] advocating that the therapist make "himself or herself transparent to the client" p. 115). The result is a *self-less* form of empathic imagination (see Meares, 1983), as in "less self, more other."

---

[5] In the 2003 movie *Freaky Friday* (Waters, 2003), a mother (Jamie Lee Curtis) and her teenage daughter (Lindsay Lohan) inadvertently come to inhabit each other's bodies for a day. They each struggle to convincingly represent the face of the other's identity while stickhandling through social realities they find both foreign and demanding.

SELF-LESS IMAGINATION

It is enough . . . to open to the ongoing process of knowing without imputing someone behind it all.
                              —Mark Epstein, Thoughts Without a Thinker (1995)

What shocks the virtuous philosopher delights the chameleon poet. . . . A poet . . . has no [unchangeable] Identity—he is continually in for and filling some other body. . . . He has no self.
                      —John Keats, The Letters of John Keats to His Family and Friends (2011)

Leo Kottke once described how playing guitar and singing on stage affects his sense of self: "Once you're out there, you disappear. . . . I don't know anything else . . . that eliminates me so readily as performance does" (Schaefer, 2007, 09:20). The poet Jane Hirshfield (1997) noted a similar sensibility arising from the "penetrating, unified, and focused" (p. 3) awareness required of poets: "In deep concentration, the self disappears. We seem to fall utterly into the object of our attention, or else vanish into attentiveness itself" (p. 4).

Mihaly Csikszentmihalyi (1990) viewed experiences such as Kottke's and Hirshfield's as instances of what he termed *flow*: "Concentration . . . so intense that there is no attention left over to think about anything irrelevant, or to worry about problems. Self-consciousness disappears, and the sense of time becomes distorted" (p. 71). Entering a flow state is possible when you possess the necessary skill to undertake an activity that you find captivating and challenging but not impossible, whether writing, dancing, gardening, rock climbing, or playing chess, sports, or music.

Although a sense of self will often dissipate as a result of your being absorbed in a captivating task, you can also reverse the order of what transpires: You can intentionally disregard the boundary of your circumscribed self to facilitate your absorbed engagement in some desired undertaking. Late one night in 1985, Bruce Springsteen and dozens of his fellow American pop luminaries—including Harry Belafonte, Bob Dylan, Ray Charles, Michael Jackson, Billy Joel, Cyndi Lauper, Huey Lewis, Kenny Loggins, Willie Nelson, Lionel Richie, Diana Ross, Paul Simon, Tina Turner, Dionne Warwick, and Stevie Wonder—came together at a Los Angeles studio to record the song "We Are the World" as a fundraiser for famine relief in Africa (We Are the World, 2024). The producer, Quincy Jones, taped a felt-tip-scribbled sign at the entrance to the studio that read, "Check your ego at the door" (see Figure 2.1). The superstars paid heed, selflessly donating their time, care, and voices to

FIGURE 2.1. Cultivating Your Self-Less Imagination

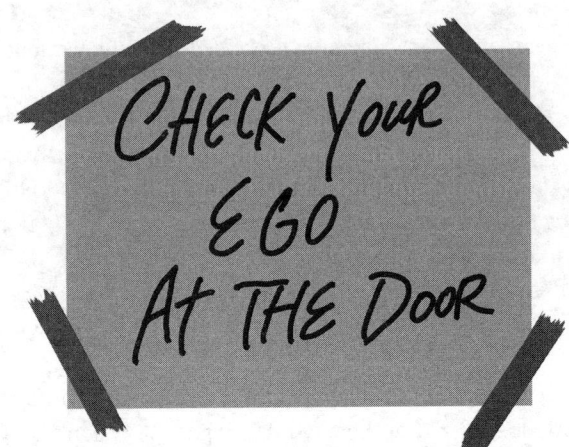

Note. This figure is based on a sign posted by Quincy Jones as a reminder to the superstar performers of "We Are the World," as depicted in the documentary *The Greatest Night in Pop* (Nguyen, 2024).

create a synergistic recording of a song that has, to date, sold more than 20 million copies.

Leaving your ego—your self—at the door is important not only for performing but also for coming to know another. Some therapists advocate a kind of "Husserlian 'phenomenological reduction' in which you . . . free [yourself] of your own self-awareness, . . . identity, and . . . preconceived notions" of the client (Mahrer, 1997, pp. 199–200). The aim is for you to be "uncontaminated, as far as possible, by [your] . . . own values, convictions, prejudices, emotional limitations, . . . and maps of healthy functioning" (Perry, 1993, p. 71). The philosopher Simone Weil believed that an understanding of the other is possible "only when we let go of our self and allow the other to grab our full attention. In order for the reality of the other's self to fully invest us, we must first divest ourselves of our own selves" (Zaretsky, 2021, p. 46). The actor Jeremy Strong commits to such divestment every time he seeks to portray another. Practicing what he calls "identity diffusion," he "clear[s] away anything—anything—that is not the character and the circumstances of the scene" (Schulman, 2021, para. 14). This necessitates "clearing away almost everything around and inside" himself so he "can be a more complete vessel for the work at hand" (Schulman, 2021, para. 14). As Bridges and

Glassman (2012) put it, "An actor empties himself of his own identity to let the role come through" (p. 106) and to ensure "there's no subject-object separation" (p. 146).

Similarly, Carl Rogers, in keeping with Theodor Reik's characterization of empathy as a process in which the therapist loses "consciousness of the self" (Lanzoni, 2018, p. 207), asserted late in his career that to empathically enter "the private perceptual world of the other" you must "lay aside your self" (Rogers, 1975, p. 4). This "lay-aside" approach to what Rogers (1975) called "an empathic way of being" unsettled Cissna and Anderson (2002), who considered it an atypical departure from his usual concern for maintaining therapists' groundedness and personal, separate uniqueness. Indeed, Cissna and Anderson explained away Rogers's "lay aside" comment as an informal, imprecise, metaphorical, and nontheoretical appeal to a lay audience.

What Cissna and Anderson (2002) saw as an unfortunate lapse, M. Friedman (1986) considered a regrettable departure from a position Rogers had taken in a public conversation with Martin Buber in 1957 (see R. Anderson & Cissna, 1997). Rogers claimed at the time that he could clearly sense the experience of the other "without losing my own personhood or separateness" (R. Anderson & Cissna, p. 30). For M. Friedman (1986), holding onto "the ground of one's own concreteness" (p. 427) is essential to avoid losing sight of yourself and your "own side of the relationship" (p. 427). You can't grasp the other in "his or her otherness" and in relationship with yourself, said M. Friedman (p. 429), if, with the goal of improving your understanding, you "bracket . . . or suspend" your awareness of yourself (p. 427).

You no doubt recognize in this critique of Rogers's supposed flip-flopping an echo of the argument over whether empathy involves the dissolution or the distinguishing of the boundary between self and other. And, as before, a resolution of the divergent positions comes into focus when you endorse the truth not of one or the other of the assertions but both at once. Lanzoni (2018) put it well: "We need the self to empathize, but we also have to leave it behind. This is one of empathy's mysteries, but it is also its promise" (p. 280). Indeed, more broadly, it is one of the mysteries and promising qualities of engaging in any flow activity. You draw on your self by accessing and implementing your personal knowledge and expertise while directing your attention outward, leaving your circumscribed self behind. This double maneuver is evident in Bruce Springsteen's experience of playing concerts. It is, he said,

> a moment of both incredible self-realization and self-erasure at the same time. You disappear and blend into all the other people that are out there and into the notes and the chords and the music that you've written. You kind of rise up and vanish into it. (Remnick, 2017, 32:41)

In Chapter 1, I described the dissolution of the self–other boundary that occurs when you're in sympathetic resonance with another person, and I explained that when you feel sympathetic concern or compassion for the person, it introduces a slight crease into your connectivity. Your caring *about* the other distinguishes you ever so slightly *from* them. I also pointed out that something analogous unfolds during mindfulness meditation. As your awareness of your breathing syncs up with your body's inhales and exhales, it dissolves the boundary between awareness and experience. But then various thoughts, sensations, and perceptions elbow their way into the midst of that connection, distracting you from the breath and disconnecting you from your focus. By turning toward and nonjudgmentally acknowledging whatever makes an appearance, you welcome it as a contribution to the whole of the meditation experience; however, the process necessarily establishes a hairline difference between your noticing and what's noticed. Your awareness is etched in bas-relief.

When you're empathically engaging with another, your sense of self becomes largely irrelevant—at least, it does when you avoid in-the-shoes style border-crossing efforts. As Fischer (2013) put it, "Empathy requires that we develop the capacity to put our own concerns aside long enough to notice what someone else is going through internally, without reference to ourselves" (p. 11). If you follow Quincy Jones's advice and intentionally check your self at the door to the therapy room, and if you then successfully get absorbed in the flow of the task (Csikszentmihalyi, 1990), you'll be well placed to send your self-less, untethered therapeutic imagination (Zaki, 2019) into their world. Nevertheless, a discrete difference is maintained between you and the client by virtue of the directionality—the relational shape—of the empathic interaction.

THE RELATIONAL SHAPE OF EMPATHY

I appl[y] . . . the term symmetric *to all those forms of interaction that could be described in terms of competition, rivalry, mutual emulation, and so on (i.e., those in which A's action of a given kind . . . stimulate B to action of the same kind, which, in turn, . . . stimulate[s] A to further similar actions). . . .*

In contrast, I appl[y] . . . the term complementary *to interactional sequences in which the actions of A and B [are] . . . different but mutually fitted [with] each other (e.g., dominance-submission, exhibition-spectatorship, dependence-nurturance).*

–Gregory Bateson, *Mind and Nature* (1979/2002, p. 180)

I made a passing reference a few pages back to the asymmetrical shape of both metaphor (Bergen, 2013) and metaphorical identity (Cohen, 2008). My imagining that "I am you" does not mean that either of us is also thereby imagining "You are me." Rather, recognizing empathy as a form of metaphorical identity makes clear that the relationship it establishes between you and your clients is nonreciprocal. In Bateson's (1979/2002) terms, empathy defines a *complementary* relationship between self and other. Each side's engagement in the dance between them is *different from* the other side's, but, like a dovetail joint, it *fits with* it (see Figure 2.2; see also Seikkula et al., 2018, p. 861).

Your empathic comments make it possible for your client to feel heard, seen, and understood. And the more you ask empathy-informed questions, the more your client responds by offering information, prompting you to pose further nuanced questions. This is how the trust and professional intimacy of a therapeutic relationship are often built. You show respect and concern and offer your developing understanding in response to the client's sharing of vulnerable details, which prompts the client's further opening up, giving rise to your subsequent, deeper understanding, and so on. The static image of the dovetail joint is limited in its ability to capture this asymmetrical pattern of empathic conversations. It is easy to see how the two contrasting parts of the joint seat into one another; however, the complementarity of the empathic relationship between you and a client can only be recognized by observing the circular feedback process of the interaction unfolding through time (represented by the arrows in Figure 2.3).

In contrast, sympathetic resonance establishes what Bateson (1979/2002) would call a *symmetrical* relationship. You and the other person are like mirror

FIGURE 2.2. The Complementary Relationship Between Therapist and Client

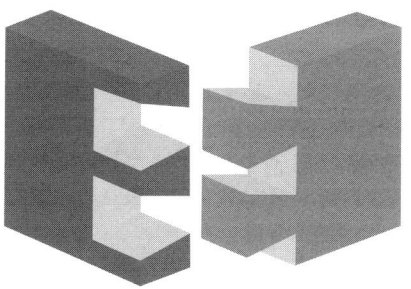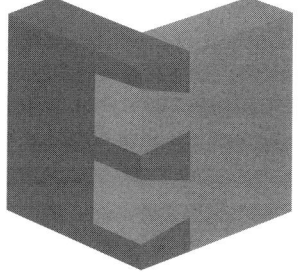

Note. Like the two sides of a dovetail joint snugging into place, the respective contributions of a therapist and client in an empathic exchange fit together not in spite of their differences but because of them.

FIGURE 2.3. The Interactive Asymmetry of Empathic Relationships

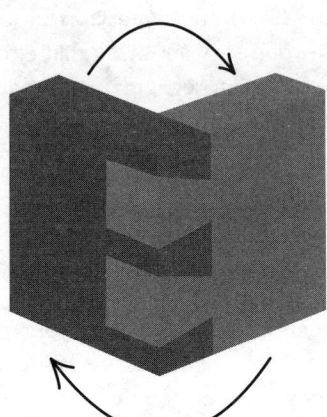

Note. The asymmetry of empathic conversations can be recognized in the circular feedback process that enjoins the differing but complementary responses and contributions of each participant.

reflections, each experiencing the same feeling. The interactive dynamic of friendship is also symmetrical: The more you ask questions about your friend's experience, the more your friend asks questions about yours. The more you dig deep to answer your friend's questions, revealing vulnerable details about your life, the more your friend reciprocates, sharing equally vulnerable details, and so on. As Figure 2.4 indicates, symmetrical interactions

FIGURE 2.4. The Interactive Symmetry of Sympathetic Resonance and Friendship-Based Relationships

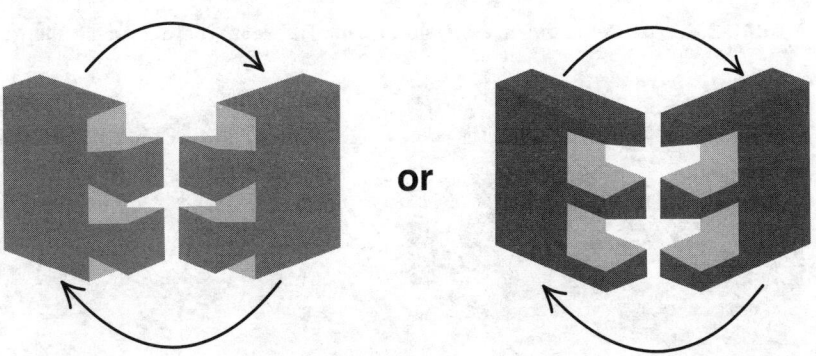

Note. The symmetry of sympathetic resonance and friendship-based relationships can be recognized in the circular feedback process that enjoins the mutual, mirrorlike reactions and/or contributions of each participant.

also unfold as circular feedback processes, creating sympathetic resonance and/or building the mutual trust and personal intimacy of friendship, one mirrored, reciprocal step at a time.

It can be difficult to grasp the inherent asymmetrical complementarity in empathic—and, more generally, compassionate and therapeutic—relationships, particularly if you, like Pema Chödrön (2001), are devoted to recognizing and honoring the intrinsic humanity and dignity of those who seek your help. She asserted that "compassion is not a relationship between the healer and the wounded" but "a relationship between equals" (Chödrön, 2001, p. 50). Carl Rogers was similarly committed to viewing his clients as equal partners in the therapeutic process, always attempting to establish an "I–Thou kind of relationship" (as cited in R. Anderson & Cissna, 1997, p. 31) with them. In a 1957 public conversation with Martin Buber, Rogers made clear that he doesn't feel different from his clients, that their ways of seeing life and experience are as valid as his, and that the therapeutic relationship is a meeting between equals (R. Anderson & Cissna; see also Rogers & Farson, 1957/2021, p. 6). He went on to describe what he saw as a fundamental symmetry—a mutuality—between the therapist and client: "It seems to me that . . . the moments where, where persons are most likely to change . . . are the moments in which perhaps the relationship is experienced the same on *both* sides" (R. Anderson & Cissna, 1997, p. 53, italic in original). This led him to speculate that "perhaps in the moments where real change takes place, then I wonder if it isn't reciprocal" (p. 62).

Buber disagreed. Earlier in the conversation, he had taken pains to illuminate the essential asymmetrical directionality—the complementarity—of therapeutic relationships:

> A man [comes] . . . to you for help. . . . The essential difference . . . between your role in this situation and his is obvious. . . . He comes for help to you. . . . You don't come to [him for] help. . . . You can . . . bodily experience his side of the situation. . . . You *feel* yourself *touched*. . . . He cannot do it at all. . . . You have . . . necessarily another attitude to the situation than he has. You are able to do something that he's not able. You are not equals and cannot be. (as cited in R. Anderson & Cissna, 1997, pp. 34–38, italic in original)

Rogers's writings have brought more clarity to the understanding and practice of empathy than anyone's; however, when it came to recognizing the relational shape of empathic and therapeutic relationships, his view was skewed by his high regard for the personhood of the client and the idea that he and the client could and should be equally changed in their therapeutic encounters. He conflated legitimacy with equality and conflated equality with mutuality, creating a blind spot that had, half a decade before his dialogue with Buber, nearly cost him his sanity.

Between 1949 and 1951, Rogers offered intensive therapy (sometimes as often as three times per week) to a client diagnosed with schizophrenia. Over the course of their work together, Rogers became convinced that he himself was "going insane": "I got to the point where I could not separate my 'self' from hers," he said. "I literally lost the boundaries of myself" (as cited in Kirschenbaum, 1979, pp. 191–192). He later concluded that "one of the worst things is for the therapist to permit the client to take over, or to be a governing influence on the therapist's life" (as cited in Baldwin, 1987, p. 31). At the end of the therapy with this client, Rogers posed the question, "If I enter, as fully as I am able, into the private world of a neurotic or psychotic individual, isn't there a risk that I might become lost in that world" (as cited in Rogers & Roethlisberger, 1952, p. 48)?

A few years later, Rogers drafted what is commonly called his as–if clause (Shlien, 1997, p. 73).[6] It served for him and since for others (e.g., Bozarth, 1997, p. 92; Hermansson, 1997, p. 140; Maibom, 2022, p. 145; Wispé, 1986, p. 318) as a bulwark against a loss of self in the midst of empathically connecting with another. To be empathic, Rogers (1959) cautioned,

> is to perceive the internal frame of reference of another . . . as if one were the person, but without ever losing the "as if" condition. Thus it means to sense the hurt or the pleasure of another as he senses it and to perceive the causes . . . as he perceives them, but without ever losing the recognition that it is *as if* I were hurt or pleased and so forth. If this "as if" quality is lost then the state is one of identification. (pp. 210–211, italic in original)

This is no doubt what Rogers had in mind the night in 1957 when he confidently told Martin Buber that he could clearly sense the client's internal experience while maintaining his own personhood (R. Anderson & Cissna, 1997, p. 30).

Challenging us to "think more complexly about empathy," Lopez (1987, p. 242) asked, "Is [Rogers's] . . . 'as–if' distinction really necessary?" Indeed, the safest protection against "losing yourself" while empathically connecting with your clients is found neither in reassuring yourself that empathy is subjunctive—as in, "it's as if I were you"—nor in continually referencing your sense of self by practicing in-your-shoes imagining and/or by making analogy-based comparisons between you and your clients. Rather, it is found one step back from your empathic efforts with each client. Your sense of self is best protected by your committing, as an empathic therapist, to safeguard the dovetail, complementary shape of your relationship with

---

[6]Rogers (1975) said he composed it sometime before 1955 (p. 3).

all clients. By eschewing symmetry in these professional encounters, you protect against the kind of boundary dissolutions (and boundary violations; see Flemons & Green, 2018) that can happen when two distinct individuals, connecting through mutual and/or reciprocal interactions, find themselves becoming "we."

Empathy can be taxing, but it needn't be harrowing or self-threatening. It requires you to take care of yourself (which I address in Chapter 3), but it won't undermine your sanity as long as you stay asymmetrically available to your clients rather than symmetrically vulnerable with them. Committing to complementarity frees you up to don your invisibility cloak and project your self-less, metaphoric imagination across the self–other divide. I have more to say about this in Chapters 4 and 5.

3 PRACTICING THERAPIST SELF-CARE

Compassionate action involves working with ourselves as much as working with others. . . .
 To relate with others compassionately . . . means not shutting down on that person, which means, first of all, not shutting down on ourselves.
—Pema Chödrön, *When Things Fall Apart* (2016)

Before we get into the nuts and bolts of putting empathic curiosity into compassionate practice, I want to pause and reflect on what this work requires of you. Learning to engage empathically is one thing; sustaining it as a therapeutic commitment, as a way of being (Rogers, 1980), is another. It requires dedication for you, day after day, to remain present for clients in their conundrums and pain—connecting with them and bearing witness to their suffering—all without pulling back, shutting down, or stressing out. Dedication is needed but so is skill. Jane Hirschfield developed an ability to stay present in trying circumstances, both as a person and as a poet, through her meditation practice:

> In any period of zazen [sitting meditation], part of what is being learned is that whatever your experience is, you can simply stay with it. You need not

https://doi.org/10.1037/0000472-004
Empathic Engagement in Clinical Practice, by D. Flemons
Copyright © 2026 by the American Psychological Association. All rights reserved.

run away. You need not be frightened. You need not reject it. Your only job is to stay on the meditation cushion and be with it and notice that eventually something will change because something always changes. And I think that was a very good instruction to me for practice, for leading my emotional life ever going forward, and for what it is that I am interested in as a poet, which is to not turn away from anything. (Shaheen, 2023, 27:25)

Not many clinicians coming into the helping professions are offered comparable training in how to take care of themselves as they rise to meet the challenge of caring about and for themselves and others.

As I discussed in Chapter 1, some clinicians attempt to cope with the emotional demands of caring by doing their utmost to avoid their own and their clients' pain. Gleichgerrcht and Decety (2012) offered several strategies for physicians to "downregulate" their sympathetic resonance (what the authors term "empathy") as protection against personal distress and resonance fatigue (which they call "compassion fatigue"). Their most radical—and surprising—suggestion was to objectify the patient: "By perceiving the [other] . . . as inhuman, the self versus other distinction increases[,] followed by a decrease in . . . [sympathetic resonance]" (which the authors call "the empathic response"; Gleichgerrcht & Decety, 2012, p. 252).

It is true that if you were to relate to patients as less than human, you could avoid being moved and, perhaps, then, negatively affected by their suffering. Zaki (2019) mentioned a study in which "individuals who dehumanized patients experienced less burnout in their work" (p. 104); however, he went on to warn of the dangers to patients of clinicians becoming callous (p. 104). As Kleinman (2019) put it, "anything that detracts from the human interaction between physicians and patients diminishes the quality, and potentially the outcome, of care" (p. 221). Considering a patient as "something less than human" neutralizes their agency (Uhrig, 2018, p. 26), and serving up "detachment with a veneer of generic tenderness communicates to the patient that the physician finds something about her emotional state either intolerable or pitiable" (Halpern, 2001, p. 25). However, dehumanization is not just a problem for patients; observational studies suggest that detachment is not a bulwark against burnout. According to Lief (2008), "the barricades we create do not help all that much; they just make things worse. We end up more fearful, less willing to extend ourselves, and stunted in our ability to express any true kindness" (p. 77).

Some of Gleichgerrcht and Decety's (2012) other suggestions, such as emotion suppression, are more widely practiced. Therapists interviewed by Besman-Albinder (2006) said that maintaining emotional distance from their clients was effective in maintaining their resilience, and Zaki (2019) noted that "disconnection can help caregivers survive their work" (p. 104). Such efforts to impose "cognitive control over autonomic responses" (Gleichgerrcht & Decety, p. 256) are in keeping with Osler's (1904) control-based strategies for remaining "imperturbable" in front of patients.

Gleichgerrcht and Decety (2012) allowed for the fact that a too robust effort to regulate "excessive caring" (p. 250) or "dampen the emotional response to suffering" (p. 255) could have an unintended rebound effect, increasing personal distress and decreasing rapport with the patient. However, I would argue that *any* effort to manhandle your feeling response has the potential to backfire, undermining your relationship with yourself and your clients (B. B. Davis, 2021). The novelist (and physician) Michael Crichton (2008) pointed out that the "human sense of self-control . . . is a user illusion. We don't have conscious control over ourselves at all. We just think we do" (p. 135). If you're caught up in this illusion, you will fail to recognize that, as Bateson (1972/2000) explained, "we do not live in the sort of universe in which simple lineal control is possible. Life is not like that" (p. 444).

Given how minds and bodies work and communicate, effective engagement with your clients will never involve keeping a snug enough but not too tight rein on your emotions. Rather than clamping down to dominate, you're far better off freeing yourself up to approbate. Of course, this means you "have to be willing to deal with pain—yours as well as theirs" (Fischer, 2013, p. 96). It isn't a matter of steeling yourself to endure it but of allowing yourself to accept it—to accept the fact of it, to accept its nuanced variability, to accept it as a doorway into connection and change.

Jon Kabat-Zinn (2023) pointed out that the root meaning of the verb *to suffer* is "to carry." With this in mind, he underscored the importance of finding "creative ways to [temporarily] put down what we are carrying . . . or [to] hold it differently" (Kabat-Zinn, 2023, p. 50). This is an excellent description of what happens in the process of empathically engaging with clients, particularly if you reverse the order of his advice. For the duration of each session, you encounter the other's suffering, but you hold it differently—not sympathetically and not just compassionately. Empathic suffering is virtual: You don't carry your clients' pain *with* or *for* them; you carry it *as* them.[1] This makes it possible at the end of the appointment for you, in keeping with Kabat-Zinn's advice, to put the suffering down, to let it go.

McIntyre et al. (2019) got it mostly right when they described empathy as a dialectic "marked by the therapist's capacity to 'feel into' the patient's

---

[1] Here, I am not referencing the third of the eight concepts that Batson (2009) distinguished as being associated with empathy: "coming to feel as another person feels" (pp. 5–6). Rather, I'm highlighting the idea of metaphorically embodying the identity of the other, of imaginatively taking on the role of being them.

emotional experience and 'feel out of' such states by regaining emotional balance" (p. 213). It is important to recognize and practice empathy as a time-bound relationship with the other, a relationship you can enter and leave. But you needn't gingerly treat empathy as a destabilizing force, a source of emotional dysregulation. It is possible to remain balanced throughout the process, not just when you come back into yourself at the end of an appointment or when you walk out of your office or the hospital at the end of the day.

Rogers (2007) believed that therapists need to be "secure enough" in themselves to ensure that they don't "get lost in what may turn out to be the strange or bizarre world of the other" (p. 3). It is essential that they're able to "comfortably return to [their] . . . own world when [they] . . . wish" (p. 3). Such security is not attained by conjuring and shielding a reified, circumscribed sense of self while venturing across the self–other threshold, nor by continually checking in with your self, using it as a referential touchstone for developing an analogy-based, in-the-shoes understanding of the person sitting across from you. Rather, as I described in Chapter 2, a sense of security derives from your willingness and ability to leave your self at the door of your therapy office as you project your untethered (Zaki, 2019), metaphoric (Cohen, 1999, 2008) imagination into the nooks and crannies of the client's embodied experience. At the end of the session, your imagination makes the return trip, heading back across the self–other boundary in the opposite direction. Coming back into yourself—collecting yourself—facilitates your leaving behind the sensory, affective, and storied details of the client's world. There is no need to carry them with you into your next session or, indeed, into your personal life.

To manage the challenges of such out-and-back journeys effectively, you need to take good care of yourself—eating and sleeping well, exercising, personally handling and responsibly resolving the intra- and interpersonal struggles that arise in day-to-day living, and actively engaging in meaningful activities with family and friends (Besman-Albinder, 2006, pp. 144–172). But also, more specifically, you need to be able to stay comfortably focused and engaged in your sessions. There is perhaps no better way of doing so than by adopting a quality of mindfulness—paying "precise attention, moment by moment, to exactly what you are experiencing, right now, separating out your reactions from the raw sensory events" (M. Epstein, 1995, p. 110).

Although mindfulness is often thought of as a form of Buddhist meditation, neither a commitment to Buddhism nor to a meditation practice is a prerequisite for developing it. Viewed from a Western, nonmeditating, social-scientific perspective (e.g., Langer, 2014), mindfulness can be understood as the "simple act of noticing new things," (Langer, n.d., para. 4) which "puts you in the present" (Langer, n.d., para. 1) and "makes you sensitive to context" (Langer, n.d., para. 1). According to Jon Kabat-Zinn (2005), who founded the secular Mindfulness-Based Stress Reduction Clinic at the UMass Medical Center in 1979, mindfulness does "not conflict with any beliefs or traditions—religious or . . . scientific—nor is it trying to sell you anything, especially not a new belief system or ideology" (pp. 6–7). He described it as a nonjudgmental way of paying attention that "nurtures greater awareness, clarity, and acceptance of present-moment reality" (Kabat-Zinn, 2005, p. 4).

You can be mindful without necessarily meditating, and you can meditate without necessarily becoming mindful, but research suggests that meditation is an effective way of learning and supporting mindfulness (K. W. Brown & Ryan, 2003, p. 843). Kabat-Zinn (1990) emphasized that the technique can "be learned and practiced . . . without appealing to Oriental culture or Buddhist authority to enrich it or authenticate it" (p. 12). True. But even if you were to turn to Buddhist sources for guidance, you would encounter not a belief system (Hagen, 2003, p. 196) but, rather, an approach to, a method for, understanding and relieving suffering—"not something to believe in but something to do" (Batchelor, 1997, p. 17). And one of those somethings is meditation. According to Chödrön (2016),

> Meditation practice is how we stop fighting with ourselves, how we stop struggling with circumstances, emotions, or moods. . . .
> This is the primary method for working with painful situations—global pain, domestic pain, any pain at all. We can stop struggling with what occurs and see its true face without calling it the enemy. . . .
> It's like inviting what scares us to introduce itself and hang around for a while. (pp. 156–157)

MINDFUL PREPARATION AND ENGAGEMENT

Some of the best elite athletes in the world—Serena Williams, Michael Jordan, Lebron James, Stephen Curry, Deena Kastor, Carli Lloyd, Christiano Ronaldo, Kobe Bryant, Tiger Woods, Bianca Andreescu (Jones, 2022)—have employed mindfulness meditation to help them prepare for high-stakes competitions (Carraça et al., 2018) and, once they're performing, to help them access and consistently return to the present-moment, mind–body coordination of being in the zone (Jackson, 2006; Mumford, 2015). Empathy isn't physically demanding, there's no competition involved, and therapy sessions are not performances. Nevertheless, therapists, like athletes, can benefit from a meditation practice to help them prepare for the unique challenges of empathically engaging with clients (McIntyre et al., 2019, p. 214) and, when they are in session, to be able to access and consistently return to the present-moment, mind–body coordination of therapeutic presence (Geller & Greenberg, 2023).

Mindful athletes don't call a timeout in the middle of a competition so they can sit down and find their breath. They instead rely on their practice-built learning to respond effortlessly to the various threats to their in-the-zone absorption. Rather than trying to shut down fear, block out inner chatter, or limit the pressure they feel to win, they maintain a foreground focus on the moment-to-moment demands of their performance while allowing potential distractions, whether from inside or outside, to move past or through them. Mindful therapists can similarly rely on what they learn in sitting meditation to help them stay present and respond noncontentiously to any internal or external challenges to their empathic engagement.

Zen teachers would say that athletes' and therapists' in-the-moment, in-the-zone presence is, itself, meditation. Zen doesn't distinguish sitting meditation (zazen) as a special activity, separate from any other mindful engagement:

> Meditation can occur anywhere. You don't have to run for a cushion. . . . Meditation is simply collecting the mind. . . . Whenever you notice that your attention is shifting away from *here* and *now*, bring it back. And when your mind checks out again, bring it back. . . . You can do this anywhere. . . . In Zen we call this meditation *practice*, because that's what we're doing: practicing the single-pointed activity of returning to *this moment*, breath by breath, day after day. (Hagen, 2003, pp. 100–101, italic in original)

You got a brief taste of mindfulness meditation in Chapter 1 when I invited you to sit in a comfortable, self-supporting posture and devote a few minutes to paying close, ongoing attention to the sensory nuances and rhythm of your breath. I encouraged you not to purposefully extend or deepen the breath but, rather, allow it to continue as is and simply attune to it so that both it and your awareness of it were moving in the same direction at the same time. In the process of such coordinated focusing, you "begin to feel your body and mind becoming synchronized. You are no longer divided" (Chödrön, 2013, p. 39).

Meditation is often physically and psychologically calming (Aylward, 2021), which both facilitates and is a common result of the development of a mind–body connection. Given how good it feels to get in sync with yourself, it isn't surprising that some people think of meditation simply as a relaxation technique. But even if you undertake it only with stress relief in mind, meditation doesn't function as the behavioral equivalent of taking a benzodiazepine. It can't be prescribed to make you relax (e.g., "Undertake two meditations and call me in the morning"). Instead, it ushers in a paradigmatically different way of relating and responding to yourself and troubled parts of your experience. Kabat-Zinn (1990) captured a sense of the difference:

> People are sent to [our] . . . [mindfulness-based] stress [reduction] clinic by their doctors because something is the matter. . . . We ask them to identify three goals that they want to work toward. . . . But then, often to their surprise, we encourage them not to try to make any progress toward their goals. . . . If one of their goals is to lower their blood pressure or to reduce their pain or their anxiety, they are instructed not to *try* to lower their blood pressure nor to *try* to make their pain or their anxiety go away. (p. 37, italic in original)

In Mary Gordon's (1998) novel *Spending*, about a successful woman painter, the protagonist's lover suggests at one point that she "try relaxing and enjoying whatever it is that's happening" (p. 130). The artist replies, "There's nothing that makes me more furious than someone telling me to Try and Relax. Try and Relax is a three-word oxymoron" (Gordon, 1998, p. 130). She understands what her partner does not: In art and life, expended effort can preclude intended effect. Mindfulness meditation helps you avoid tripping yourself up by inviting you to direct your attention not toward striving for a desired future feeling or state but toward tuning into, acknowledging, and letting go of present-moment experience, regardless of what it is.

There are several excellent phone apps (e.g., Calm, Happier, Headspace, Smiling Mind, Waking Up) that can help you get a mindfulness meditation practice up and running (okay, up and sitting); however, I suggest you not become overly reliant on the guided meditations that the apps plentifully supply. Having a pleasant, encouraging voice in your ear can help support you in your commitment to protect a few minutes to connect with yourself, and it provides an excellent foreground point of reference for keeping distractions at bay. But short-term benefits become long-term liabilities if you mistakenly believe that such guidance is necessary because you're too scattered to meditate on your own. Such an assumption would be a mistake.

If you bring just app-less you to the process of meditating, rhythmically syncing up your breath and your awareness of it, your in-the-zone, undivided concentration won't last long—maybe only just a few nanoseconds (D. Harris & Warren, 2017, p. 6). This is true for everyone. Before you know it, your concentration will be interrupted and your focus hijacked by a thought, feeling, worry, memory, perception, sensation, and/or anticipation that elbows its way onto the screen of your awareness. Rather than trying to arm up—or app up—against it, you can simply and nonjudgmentally make "a soft mental note" (Goldstein, 2002, p. 94) of whatever ephemeral mind–body snarl or sparkle is grabbing you and then turn your attention back to your breath. Instead of effortfully attempting to retain your point of focus, you allow for the inevitability of losing it and the ever-present opportunity to

> **BOX 3.1**
> **AN EXPERIENCE OF MINDFULNESS MEDITATION**
>
> Sitting comfortably, with your eyes open or closed, bring your attention to the rhythm of your breathing. As you focus in, you may notice that your breath feels somewhat self-consciously awkward for a little while. Don't worry—that will diminish. Track the movement of air, in and out, by attending to sensations in your nostrils, chest, abdomen, or back, and then notice how these sensations change as the air, now warmed by the inside of your body, is released. The rate and depth of your breath is fine just as it is; you don't need to purposefully slow or deepen it. When something about it changes, just stay with it. Match the trajectory of your awareness with the trajectory of your breath so they're like a couple of synchronized swimmers, mirroring each other.
>
> Before you know it, something will steal your attention away from your breath, right from under your nose. One moment you're right there, with your breath in foreground focus—in . . . out . . . in—and the next moment, you're immersed in hoping, grousing, wincing, wondering, planning, fretting, recalling, or regretting, and your breath is out of sight and out of mind.
>
> And then, out of the blue, you realize that your awareness got sidetracked. You acknowledge the detour, let go of whatever has been captivating you, and without judgment or disgruntlement, you bring your breath back into foreground focus—the moving, sensory, present-moment quality of it—and, following it, you're back, for a time, in sync.

effortlessly return to it (Lindsay & Creswell, 2019). Indeed, "if you have to let go of distractions and begin again thousands of times, fine. That's not a roadblock to the practice—that *is* the practice" (Salzberg, 2011, p. 50). In Box 3.1, I offer you a taste of what it looks and feels like.

Different traditions and different teachers within each vary somewhat in the suggestions they offer for undertaking a mindfulness meditation practice,[2]

---

[2] If you'd like to find out more about undertaking a mindfulness meditation practice, I can recommend some practical books to help you get started: Pema Chödrön's (2013) *How to Meditate*; Bhante Gunaratana's (2011) *Mindfulness in Plain English*; Dan Harris's (2014) *Ten Percent Happier*; Dan Harris and Jeff Warren's (2017) *Meditation for Fidgety Skeptics*; Sam Harris's (2014) *Waking Up*; John Kabat-Zinn's (1990) *Full Catastrophe Living* and (2005) *Wherever You Go, There You Are*; Jack Kornfield's (2004) *Meditation for Beginners*; Matthieu Ricard's (2010) *Why Meditate?*; and Sharon Salzberg's (2011) *Real Happiness*.

but all generally agree that over the course of 5 to 30 minutes of daily sitting, you can expect to (a) focus on the rhythm of your breathing; (b) lose this focus when more compelling items of experience draw your attention; (c) come to recognize the loss of focus; (d) gratefully acknowledge this recognition because it makes it possible to (e) let go of the distraction and to (f) nonjudgmentally refocus on, and get back in sync with, the breath; and (g) continue cycling in this way throughout your sitting.

Some version of this process provides athletes with what they need to show up and stay in the zone; likewise, it can give you the necessary focusing skill to collect yourself before, after, and/or during breaks between seeing clients. However, you face unique, intra- and interpersonal demands when working empathically with people who are suffering. You need to be able to comfortably protect yourself for imaginative excursions into the world of the other without an inadvertent hardening of the boundaries—without resorting to defining and defensively guarding a reified sense of self. To deftly manage such a balancing act, you may find it helpful to augment your practice.

My paternal grandfather immigrated to Canada from England early in the 20th century. I still remember his teaching me and my brothers how to alter or enhance the trajectory of a billiard or table tennis ball by adding spin to it—by, as he said at the time, "putting a little mustard" or "putting a little English" on it. You can similarly put a little mustard or a little English on your practice of mindfulness meditation by introducing different imaginative spins to the process. I offer three: collecting and releasing, sending and receiving, and including and learning.

Collecting and Releasing

The first imagination-enhanced method offers a nonadversarial way of preparing for and responding to mind–body overload by drawing in and releasing mind–body ephemera (e.g., emotions, senses, thoughts, stress) with your breath (see Box 3.2). By doing this, you develop your ability to later implement this drawing in and releasing as a behind-the-scenes, automatic skill if, for example, you find yourself in the middle of an appointment feeling overwhelmed. Rather than distancing from the client or attempting to control what you're feeling, you can simply allow whatever is grabbing hold of you to dissipate with each easy exhale. You mindfully engage with yourself in meditation to develop the capacity to mindfully and empathically engage with clients in session. Such a practice can help prepare you for in-the-moment handling of your affective experience during the session (cf. McIntyre et al., 2019, p. 214).

> **BOX 3.2**
> **AN EXPERIENCE OF COLLECTING AND RELEASING**
>
> As you begin meditating and you attune to your breath, imagine that, as your lungs are drawing in oxygen, they're also drawing in and collecting, from throughout your mind and body, the ephemeral thoughts, images, sensations, tensions, and/or feelings that are competing for your attention. (It helps to recognize that they're all ephemeral, even the ones that seem entrenched.) And then on the next breath out or the one after that—no hurry—imagine the easy release of carbon dioxide being coupled with the easy release of the mind-body ephemera that your lungs have collected. No need to expend any effort; you aren't forcibly expelling anything. Your exhale is occasioned by the relaxing of your diaphragm and muscles in your chest, allowing CO_2 and thoughts, CO_2 and images, CO_2 and sensations, CO_2 and tensions, CO_2 and feelings to be effortlessly released into the atmosphere.
>
> Not long after you institute this circular process, some idea, worry, or scenario will elude collection. Instead of getting drawn into your lungs, it will draw your attention into it, stealing your awareness away from your breath and away from your intention to gather and release, along with your breath, anything that's not your breath. It will hold your attention in its thrall until, at some point, your awareness, instead of being captivated by this captor, is released from its grip. Able now to recognize and acknowledge the capture for what it was and this moment of freedom for what it is—a release!—your awareness can return to the breath. On your next inhale, the story of what just transpired can itself be effortlessly collected, and on the exhale, without agitation or recrimination, carried by the current of air exiting your lungs, it can be effortlessly released into the atmosphere.

Receiving and Sending

A second way of adding imaginative spin to your mindful preparation is to undertake an adaptation of *tonglen* meditation, the Tibetan Buddhist compassion practice of "sending and receiving" that I introduced in Chapter 1 (see Box 3.3 for an example of how to put this into practice). You may remember that this method provides a way of learning how not to turn away from the other's suffering, not to recoil from it, not to hold it at arm's length, not to numb yourself to it. You reverse the usual way of handling pain. "Instead of taking in what we desire and rejecting what we do not, we take

> **BOX 3.3**
> ### AN EXPERIENCE OF RECEIVING AND SENDING
>
> Begin as you would any mindfulness meditation. Find a comfortable position to sit and, if you leave your eyes open, a comfortable spot to rest your gaze. Attune to the sensory qualities of your breath so when you're breathing in, you know you're breathing in, and when you're breathing out, you know you're breathing out (Goldstein, 2016, p. 50).
>
> When you're ready, imagine a person sitting in front of you, a client in the throes of suffering. Pairing your imagination with your breath, envision on the next inhale that you're drawing the other's pain into your body, receiving it. Welcome it in, feeling, acknowledging, embracing it. You might picture how it looks as you inhale it, or you may imagine more the idea of it or the visceral feel of it as it comes into your lungs. Or perhaps you'll be able to both see and feel it, or you'll get both an idea and a tangible sense of it.
>
> And then, in the same way you rely on your body to convert the food you swallow into the nutrients that energize and repair your cells, you can imagine your body distilling the received suffering into essential component elements and converting and combining these into "lightness, ease, [and] peacefulness" (Fischer, 2013, p. 34). On your exhale, imagine sending out this transmuted pain as a "healing light" (p. 35), bathing the other in its glow, or perhaps as an invisible mist of well-being that the client can breathe in.
>
> Continue coordinating this imagined transmutation with your respiration for the duration of the meditation. All the pain you take in on the inhale is digested, distilled, converted, and then, on the exhale, released as relief and a fine-tuned source of healing.

in what we have rejected and send out what we desire—basically the opposite of 'normal'" (Lief, 2008, p. 72). You welcome in the other's suffering, and in your imagination, you transmute it. According to Lindsay and Creswell (2019), "Acceptance is thought to transform how momentary experiences are observed and processed, facilitating engagement (i.e., welcoming in) and subsequent disengagement (i.e., letting go) with emotional stimuli, and thus enriching experience while also reducing emotional reactivity" (p. 2).

Although this meditation is ostensibly organized as a means of offering compassion to an imagined other, it also offers a vehicle for practicing what Neff (2012) described as self-compassion. As I discussed in Chapter 1, all compassion practices are grounded in the notion that if you fully absorb the realization that we all suffer, the distinction between self and other becomes an arbitrary divide, particularly when you're actively engaged in offering a healing response. Thus, a compassionate response to the suffering of another, in some sense, folds you, yourself, into its embrace, and an appreciation and expression of self-compassion is a point of departure into feeling compassion for all others. Each is a tributary to the other.

I also think of tonglen meditation as a condensed, body-grounded analog of what unfolds more gradually between you and your clients during the entire therapeutic process. In therapy, you welcome in—you "receive"—your clients' descriptions and expressions of pain, and you respond with—you "send"—compassionate care, empathic curiosity, and therapeutic invitations for change. Such an accepting and heartfelt responsiveness contributes to alterations and transformations of clients' experiences. In your tonglen meditation, you practice such receptivity and creative resourcefulness in the face of suffering, one breath at a time.[3]

You won't have the attentional bandwidth to actively undertake this imagined exchange while in conversation with your clients, but you may find it helpful to turn to it during pauses or periods of engaged silence. And, just as you bring a practiced mindfulness into your sessions with clients, you can also bring a practiced tonglen sensibility—a commitment to the transmutation of suffering—that supports you in staying present and engaged throughout each appointment.

Including and Learning

A third way of putting a little English on your meditation practice begins by turning toward and responding warmly to whatever shows up on your screen of awareness: "It all just gets included. . . . There's nothing outside of the practice. Whatever arises can be included. . . . In essence, nothing is a distraction, because everything can be included" (Goldstein, 2020, 01:06; Box 3.4 offers an example of how to do this). This commitment to inclusion is reflected in a poem by the 13th-century Sufi poet Rumi:[4]

> This being human is a guest house.
> Every morning a new arrival.
> A joy, a depression, a meanness,

---

[3]For more on tonglen, see Pema Chödrön's (2016) *When Things Fall Apart*, Norman Fischer's (2013) *Trainings in Compassion*, and/or Dzigar Kongtrul's (2016) *The Intelligent Heart*.

[4]The translation of Rumi's "The Guest House" is copyrighted © 1994 by Coleman Barks. Reprinted with permission from Coleman Barks.

some momentary awareness comes
as an unexpected visitor.
Welcome and entertain them all! (Barks, 1994, p. 109)

The meditation teacher Jeff Warren (n.d.) brings an analogous attitude of invitational warmth to a guided meditation he calls "Welcome to the Party":

> The whole principle of this "Welcome to the party" meditation is that everything and everyone is welcome. . . . You are an affable host. "So happy to see you," you might say, "Welcome to the party of my direct experience." . . . Make this your mantra: Welcome the insistent thought, welcome the annoying sensation, welcome the distracting sound. There are no enemies in this meditation, no problems—only new things to notice and to welcome.

BOX 3.4

AN EXPERIENCE OF INCLUDING AND LEARNING

Go ahead and begin this meditation like the others, sitting comfortably, resting your gaze or closing your eyes, and syncing your awareness with your breath.

Now, be on the lookout for sources of annoyance, distress, or pain. Regardless of whether they arrive from outside (an uncomfortable temperature, an unpleasant smell, a too-loud television in the next room) or inside (a jabbing or aching sensation, a critical voice in your head, a queasy feeling), find and focus for a moment on one that in any other circumstance you'd do your best to block, diminish, or fix.

Imagine holding the discomfort in your hands, gently but securely, and however counterintuitive it might seem, welcome it into your awareness. Bring it in close so you can discern and unravel the details of it, and breathe into or through it as a way of tolerating and relaxing into its presence, deepening your capacity to continue bearing witness. Take careful account not only of the particularities of your perceptions but also your reactions to what you notice—how you register the presence of whatever it is that you're at odds with, as well as how you're reacting to it. Derive, as best you can, a felt sense (Gendlin, 1981) of the intensity and valence of the experience, as well as a granular appreciation of the thoughts and affect that are stirred into it. In the process, you will gain fluency in the intrapersonal communications involved in experiences such as loss, pain, shock, desire, distress, surprise, expectation, clinging, ignoring, confusion, avoidance, obsession, resentment, disappointment, and so on. Explore them as an absorbed observer committed to grasping their inner workings, their logic. In other words, connect with yourself empathically.

Included, welcomed, and then what? As with the first mustard-added modification to your meditation practice, you could always just imagine collecting and then releasing whatever you've welcomed in. Or, in keeping with the second way of adding spin, before sending back out whatever you've collected and welcomed, you could imagine transmuting it into some kind of healing light or substance. But there's a third alternative: Rather than releasing or transmuting what you've included, you can bear witness to it, turn to it with warm curiosity, and treat it as an opportunity for learning.

When you can bear witness to your discomfort in this way, tolerating it and learning from it, you have a valuable resource to bring with you into sessions with clients. In Chapter 2, I described how your sympathetic resonance with clients can help inform your empathic imagination (e.g., Geller & Greenberg, 2023); however, your internally sourced experience can contribute valuable information, as well.

According to Lisa Feldman Barrett, emotions are stories the brain tells about our affective arousal (Huberman, 2023). Emotions are the instantaneous sense we make of what we're feeling; as such, they are interpretations influenced by personal history, expectation, and context. When the context is a therapy session with a distressed client, it becomes possible to turn with curiosity toward difficult feelings welling up in you as a source of potential insight, not just about you, necessarily, but also about the other person. If you get skilled at tolerating and listening to your internal misgivings and murmurings, they can become potentially enriching and animating contributions to your understanding of the client rather than annoying and problematic roadblocks to it.

Incorporating Imagination-Enhanced Mindfulness Meditation Into Clinical Practice

Let's test drive how a mindfulness meditation practice and the three added-mustard modifications can help you stay present and empathically connect with clients, even in high-stakes situations. Imagine you're just starting your career, having just completed all requirements for licensure. Today, you're 20 minutes into a first session with an edgy, isolated, sometimes-tearful client who, on the intake form, mentioned being hospitalized several months ago following a suicide attempt. She seems caught in a doom cycle of loss, despair, and hopelessness.

If you're like many therapists, you will, at least to some extent, sympathetically resonate with the client, registering her turmoil in your gut or chest. Feeling concerned about and responsible for the client's safety, your brain will likely trigger the release of the hormones adrenaline and noradrenaline (epinephrine and norepinephrine) to help you physiologically prepare to meet the demands of the situation. As a result, you may feel jittery, with your voice a little shaky, your mouth a little dry, and/or your palms a little damp.

If, wanting to appear calm and professional, you make an anxious attempt to stifle physical indicators of anxiety, you can get caught up in a self-reflective loop or escalating spiral. Responding to the demands of the situation (the attempt to shut down what you're feeling), your brain may trigger the release of more of the very hormones responsible for the sensations you're attempting to squelch, thereby prolonging or even heightening your discomfort. Such efforts will also steal precious attention from your engagement with the client, making it all the more difficult for the two of you to connect.

Enter mindfulness. It may help to recognize that your body sensations are not a sign of something being wrong with you but are, rather, an indicator of your brain's and body's effort to help you rise to the challenges you're facing. But just as—or more—important will be your ability to acknowledge and let go of sensations and thoughts as they come into your awareness, nonjudgmentally bringing your attention back each time to the therapeutic conversation. You can implement with your clients a skill you develop in sitting meditation:

> When you are practicing zazen, do not try to stop your thinking. Let it stop by itself. If something comes into your mind, let it come in, and let it go out. It will not stay long. When you try to stop your thinking, it means you are bothered by it. Do not be bothered by anything. It appears as if something comes from outside your mind, but actually it is only the waves of your mind, and if you are not bothered by the waves, gradually they will become calmer and calmer. (Suzuki, 2006, p. 22)

If you were to put some collecting-and-releasing spin onto this mindful engagement, you would, in the background, imagine your inhales drawing still inchoate thoughts and sensations into your lungs before they interrupt your focus and then effortlessly breathing them out. Adding a receiving-and-sending spin would inspire you to warmly welcome and embrace both the client's and your own distress as fuel for the healing light you imagine illuminating your session. And putting a little including-and-learning mustard onto your mindful engagement would introduce the possibility of utilizing your "discomfort as an empathic steppingstone into the subjective experience of the client" (Flemons & Gralnik, 2013, p. 64).

You can thus use the valence and intensity of what's going on within you to flesh out and viscerally nuance your emotional imagination of the client's world, animating and providing dimensionality to your empathic curiosity. This doesn't mean that what you come to understand—what you imagine—will necessarily be accurate. That can only be determined by garnering feedback from the client as you tentatively offer your developing empathic sensibility. Critical details about how the client is orienting to and making sense of their circumstances might come into focus only by virtue of how they contrast with what you anticipated they might be, given your affective turmoil. I return to this point in the next chapter.

MINDFUL DISENGAGEMENT

Empathy is not a state of being but a choice to engage (Jamison, 2014, p. 23; Zaki, 2014), a compassionate commitment to bring interpersonal curiosity and body-assisted knowing into your relationship with clients. If you're going to learn how to empathically feel your way into another's experience (the focus of the next two chapters), it is essential to know first how to transition out of it, how to disengage from the connection. Actors face a similar challenge. Of course, empathizing with a client requires different skills from those involved in depicting a character on the stage or screen. Nevertheless, both kinds of engagement involve imaginatively crossing the self–other boundary without bringing a sense of self along for the ride, imaginatively embodying the story and experience of someone other, and then, at some point, bringing the imaginative excursion to a close by reconstituting both the boundary and a sense of personal identity. It is only safe to self-lessly undertake such transformations if you're fully able to come back into yourself when the situation warrants it and whenever your well-being requires it (Meares, 1983).

Some movie and television actors, committed to verisimilitude, have focused their attention primarily on the ingress (the embodiment) part of their character portrayals, neglecting the egress part of the process—the need for an exit plan, for getting out of character, for "de-roling" (Garville, n.d.). Zaki (2019) described the lengths to which Adrien Brody went in the movie *The Pianist* to capture the desperation and integrity of a Jewish musician and composer hiding out in the Warsaw Ghetto during the Holocaust. Brody "ended his relationship, disconnected his phones, and moved to Europe. He spent months alone, playing the piano for hours each day and eating so little that he shed forty pounds" (Zaki, 2019, p. 78). He later regretted going to such extremes, which resulted in posttraumatic stress disorder and an eating disorder (Sharf, 2024). Daniel Day-Lewis, playing a character who wastes away of a heart ailment in *The Last of the Mohicans*, similarly starved himself (Schulman, 2021), and during the filming of *My Left Foot*, where he played a person with cerebral palsy, Day-Lewis refused to get out of the character's wheelchair while on set or even during breaks (Crumlin, 2021, para. 11). By holding himself in a hunched-over position for weeks of filming, he cracked two ribs (Crumlin, 2021).

This uninterrupted, total immersion approach to acting is also practiced by Jeremy Strong, the actor I mentioned in Chapter 2. He starred in the television series *Succession* (Armstrong, 2018–2023), playing the tortured son, Kendall Roy, of a domineering patriarch, Logan Roy. Strong stayed in role, even when the cameras were off, relating to other performers in the production as if they, too, were characters, not colleagues. The classically trained British stage actor Brian Cox, who played Logan, publicly expressed both irritation with and concern for Strong's method: "I just worry about what he does to himself. I worry about the crises he puts himself through in order to prepare" (Schulman, 2021, para. 21). Cox, who takes a "turn it on, turn it off" approach to acting, considers it unhealthy not to be able to "separate yourself off while you're doing the job" (Schulman, 2021, para. 21).

A blurring between the actor's sense of self and the character being performed can result in the actor's personal life "supplant[ing] the character in performance. . . . Conversely, the actor's character may take over offstage, with the actor carrying over character behavior into everyday life. A consequence of both processes may be emotional distress" (Burgoyne et al., 1999, p. 11, as cited in Maxwell et al., 2015, p. 71). This concern was confirmed by Taylor (2017), whose research revealed that many students at the leading drama schools in Australia were suffering from extreme moods and personal difficulties as a result of not protecting the necessary time and space for adequately separating themselves from their roles. Their symptoms of what Seton (2008) called "post-dramatic stress" reflect a bias in acting schools toward helping actors take on challenging roles without providing enough, if any, guidance for how to "remove" a role or debrief after one or more performances.

Elizabeth Debicki, the Australian actor who played Princess Diana for two seasons on the Netflix series *The Crown*, is a case in point. She spent a year researching and preparing for the role, altering the register of her voice (Davies, 2024) and "perfecting Diana's specific dialect and cadence," as well as her "gait and gestural language" (Soloski, 2023, para. 11). Approaching acting as "blurring the real life [of the character] and the imaginary" (Soloski, 2023, para. 12), she found that Diana's mannerisms "ingrained so deeply" into herself, she continued unintentionally emulating the princess for a long while after the series ended (Davies, 2024, para. 4). A year after filming had wrapped, she described herself as still "a bit emotionally stuck in," saying, "I don't really think I've left" (Soloski, 2023, para. 21). The actor Larry Parks experienced something similar in preparing for and filming *The Jolson Story*. "Parks became [Al] Jolson to a point of which he was a little frightened. He could not stop being Jolson . . . even when he was alone" (Lanzoni, 2018, p. 213).

Therapists analogously risk suffering from "postempathic stress" if they don't know how to manage their sympathetic resonance with clients or how to release their embodied imagination of their clients' experiences. The psychologist Eric Greenleaf once saw a therapist in his practice whose unbounded resonance with a schizophrenic patient had resulted in the therapist developing some of the patient's frightening symptoms (E. Greenleaf, personal communication, December 12, 2022). She told Eric she wasn't sure she could continue working. Eric talked with her about how chefs are able to get an in-depth appreciation of the flavor profile of their dishes without actually eating them. They simply dip in a finger or spoon once or twice and use taste, rather than ingestion, to guide their sense of what needs to be adjusted or added. This metaphor became an organizing principle for the therapist's learning how to manage professional empathic relationships.

Some years ago, a young psychiatrist, Audrey, reached out to me with a similar postempathic stress problem. She had, she said, "become infected" by some of her patients' symptoms, including panic attacks, compulsive hand washing, and intrusive, perseverating thoughts (cf. Shotter, 2005, p. 137, who noted that all of us, when we interact with others, are "'infected', so to speak, with the 'otherness' of the other"). Distraught at not being able to maintain her autonomy and horrified by how "crazy" she felt, Audrey was seriously questioning her choice of specialty. She described herself as an "empath,"[5] someone who had always "picked up on the vibes" of the people around her. In fact, she said, precisely this sensitivity had initially inspired her to go into medicine and then pursue a 4-year residency in psychiatry. But because her sympathetic resonance (what she called "empathy") didn't come "with an off-switch," her heartfelt efforts to improve the well-being of her patients were taking a significant toll on her own.

To help make it safe for Audrey to continue in her profession, I introduced her to mindfulness meditation, as well as to some of the engagement techniques I discuss in Chapter 5; however, the first thing we did was to create a simple ritual for her to physically and symbolically usher herself back into an autonomous sense of self. I remarked that Audrey's urge to wash her hands was an inspired response to her feeling infected by her patients. Noting that

---

[5]In Chapter 1, I explained why the more appropriate designation would be *sympath*; however, I didn't talk to Audrey about her word choice.

primary care physicians assiduously employ this procedure between physical exams to protect themselves and their patients from illness, I asked if she would be willing to readopt a safety procedure she'd learned in med school. She agreed to take a quick trip to the bathroom between sessions, during which time she would methodically use soap and water, even for just a few seconds, to efficiently and fully rinse away the previous patient's suffering. This and the subsequent drying of her hands would serve as a tangible point of focus for literally getting back in touch with her personhood before seeing the next patient. I then suggested that she make one last trip to the sink at the end of the day to ensure that any lingering patient symptoms were safely washed down the drain before she headed home. Milton Erickson (2008a) would have classified my suggestion as a form of *utilization*. Instead of orienting toward helping Audrey contain or control her compulsion to wash her hands, I put it to good therapeutic use, rendering it legitimate and helpful in resolving her struggles (see Flemons, 2020, 2022).

With her washing compulsion therapeutically retrofitted as a mindful ritual for coming back into herself, Audrey had a reliable, symbolically meaningful method for disentangling from her patients. This became the first step in developing a "turn it on, turn it off" approach to boundary management in her empathic connections. As we continued working together, her "infection" symptoms faded away, and as she was able to reclaim her identity, her feelings of vulnerability decreased significantly.

Small rituals or routines can serve as mind–body transportation devices, ferrying people from problematic to resourceful ways of relating to self, others, and circumstances. Some athletes employ rituals to prepare for competition (involving what they wear, eat, chant), and some activate behavioral routines when they need, mid-game, to get in—or back in—the zone, such as symbolically dispatching an error they've just made by wiping their hand on their uniform or a piece of equipment (Karageorghis, 2008). Others perform a distinct patterned movement in preparation for, say, the next serve, stroke, pitch, free throw, or penalty shot—bouncing or turning a ball; tapping or turning a racquet, club, stick, or bat; adjusting a hat or piece of clothing. For example, throughout her career, Serena Williams would, before her first serve, consistently bounce the tennis ball five times and, before her second, two times (Norton, 2024, p. 54). During the 2024 Women's National Basketball Association season, before each of her 56 free throws, Caitlin Clark would first touch her shoes, then pat her chest, take a deep breath, and rehearse the shot (Phelps, 2024).

Taylor (2017) described several purposeful steps actors can take to de-role, "leaving their characters in the dressing room" ("How to De-role" section), including the use of the imagination (visualization), the body (singing, movement), and mind-altering techniques (deep breathing and meditation). Undertaking the steps as a consciously performed ritual infuses it with symbolic significance, assisting in the demarcation of the actor and character. Rituals include leaving behind a talisman that is exclusively carried during performing (Taylor, 2017), mindfully placing the character's props back on the props table, removing and hanging up the character's costume, physically shaking the character off, and washing away the character in the shower, aided by using soap of a specific scent (perfume or cologne) that the actor associates with the character and only wears during the performance (Gardiner et al., n.d.).

Rituals work as transportation devices because they conjure a context for identity change—for shifts in your mind–body relationship to your self, the other, and your circumstances. You may find it helpful to invent a brief, mindfully performed ritual to carry out between each of your therapy sessions (and again at the end of the day), one that symbolically disperses your empathic connection with your last client and puts you in touch with a grounded sense of yourself as you prepare to engage with the next one. The procedure needn't be elaborate and needn't involve a tennis ball, talisman, or a scent or costume change. But you might draw inspiration from athletes, who know a thing or two about what it takes to be fully present in the moment, and from actors, who need to know how to leave the self behind for a time and, later, how to reclaim it.

R. Epstein (2017), a family physician, described what he does to show up for every patient he sees:

> Over the years I have developed a habit of pausing momentarily before entering any patient's room. With my hand on the doorknob, I quietly take a breath to help me become more present in preparation for the visit—I mentally set aside everything that has happened with the patient I have just finished seeing and other events of the day so that I can be fresh and available. I let go of expectations. It takes just a second or two. (p. 64)

The ritual itself can become its own talisman, a touchstone reminder or context marker (Bateson, 1972/2000, pp. 289–290) for symbolically evoking an unencumbered freedom to move, breathe, and disentangle. Offering an efficient, mind–body means of refreshing and regrouping also sets the stage for you to fire up your curiosity and compassionate commitment to make a difference. You're ready, once again, to empathically engage. But to do so effectively, you need to attend to how you're orienting to the client.

4 ORIENTING EMPATHICALLY TO CLIENTS

Wonder . . . is the hinge between ignorance and knowledge.
—Jerome A. Miller, *Wonder As Hinge* (1989, p. 53)

Several years ago, a mother, Jeanine, contacted the training clinic for my university's family therapy program, requesting a session for herself and her 11-year-old son, Cody, whose father had recently died. Cody, she said, was agitated and impatient with her and was balking at going to school or seeing his friends. Concerned about how isolated and withdrawn he was, Jeanine hoped a therapist could get through to him so he could give voice to his grief. The case was assigned to my practicum team of six students, and I chose one of them, Randall, to be the lead therapist. He would work with the mother and son in front of a one-way mirror while I and the rest of the team watched from the observation room behind it.

    Before heading to the waiting room to greet the family, Randall met with the team for a brief presession consultation. He said he was confident he could connect well with Cody because he himself had lost his father when he was about the same age. I cautioned him to avoid bringing his personal history into the conversation, but my concerns didn't register. As Randall saw

---

https://doi.org/10.1037/0000472-005
Empathic Engagement in Clinical Practice, by D. Flemons
Copyright © 2026 by the American Psychological Association. All rights reserved.

it, the pain from his tragic loss had started him on the path to where he was now, pursuing an advanced degree in a helping profession. He was proud of how it had shaped his professional identity, and he saw an opportunity to now shine a light for someone who desperately needed it. Off he went to collect his clients.

The session derailed almost immediately. Randall asked Jeanine what had brought them in and what they hoped to get out of therapy. She explained the circumstances of her husband's untimely death and described how devastated and disoriented she and her son had been since. She'd been fine with Cody staying home from school the first few days after the funeral, but now, more than another week had passed, and they were fighting every morning about his needing to get back to class. More often than not, she lost the battle; her nerves were too jangled to persist in trying to convince him. Most of the day, he stayed barricaded in his room playing video games.

Randall proclaimed himself to be a video game enthusiast also and then, turning to Cody, leaned forward and said reassuringly, "My dad died of cancer when I was 12, so I understand how painful this is for you."

"No, you don't!" Cody retorted. "Nobody does."

Taken aback, Randall patiently reassured him, "No, really, I actually *do*. I went through it myself, so I totally get it. It was the hardest thing I've ever faced. I didn't want to go to school either. I didn't want to see my friends, play sports—for a while there, quite a while, actually, nothing mattered."

Cody seethed, "You don't understand a *thing*," and closed up, refusing to engage for the rest of the session. He and his mother didn't return for a second appointment.

Randall's efforts at empathy went sideways for three interconnected reasons, all having to do with how he undertook the challenge of establishing a therapeutic alliance with his client (Norcross & Lambert, 2018). He approached empathy as a relationship of mutual vulnerability, held tight to a misguided certainty about what he knew, and took for granted that claiming he understood his client's experience would prove that he did. This chapter details five orienting commitments for empathic engagement—eschewing mutuality, embracing ignorance, not presuming, not judging, and not claiming—that, if you adopt them, can help you orient empathically without inadvertently alienating the people with whom you wish to connect.

ESCHEWING MUTUALITY

Is complementarity always somehow better than symmetry?
—Gregory Bateson, *Steps to an Ecology of Mind* (1972/2000, p. 336)

In the sixth episode of the sixth season of the television series *This is Us* (S. K. Watson et al., 2022), a young ballet dancer, Stacey, performs a solo in the autumn showcase of her dance school (NBC, 2022). The stakes are high because recruiters from major dance companies are in the audience. Early on, Stacey is greeted by enthusiastic applause as she executes a stunning series of back-to-back pirouettes, but just then, she loses her balance and falls. The audience gasps and sits in stunned silence. Stacey remains slumped on the stage but looks over to one of the main characters of the series, Beth, a former prima ballerina and now the recruitment director for the school, who has been standing in the wings. Beth walks out onto the stage and kneels beside the young dancer. "Are you hurt?" she asks.

"I don't think so," Stacey whispers.

"Okay, let's get you up" (28:42).

Stacey tells her she can't and, clearly humiliated, apologizes for letting Beth down, along with everyone else. Beth takes this in and then divulges a painful moment from her past: "You know, when I was dancing, I fell. It was a bigger kind of fall. Bigger than this. I felt so alone" (28:58). She goes on to tell Stacey that she'll sit with her on the stage until the audience gets bored and leaves. "Or," she offers, "You can get up. You can start again. And I'll be waiting for you right off stage after you take your bow" (29:28). Stacey collects herself, takes it from the top, performs brilliantly, and this being television, later goes on to land the lead role in a performance of the Nutcracker with the Houston Ballet.

In Chapter 2, I distinguished between the symmetrical mutuality of sympathy and the dovetail complementarity of empathy, and I explained that in sympathy-defined affective relationships, trust and mutual understanding are built through comparable displays of vulnerability. Beth's offering up the story of her own fall established a sympathetic resonance with Stacey's, granting her the requisite standing to successfully challenge and inspire the young dancer to lift herself up by her own pointe-shoe ribbons. The narrative arc of their interaction follows the logic of mutuality typically seen in friendships.

Given the symmetrical shape of sympathetic resonance, it isn't surprising that inside the offering of mutual vulnerability, sharing can sometimes take on a competitive edge. Beth didn't say that her fall was just as devastating as Stacey's; she proclaimed that it was worse. If, in real life, someone like Beth were to offer this kind of message to someone like Stacey, it would not, I suspect, be so warmly and gratefully received. This is borne out in a story I share later in this chapter about a friend and her sister.

If you and I were friends, your willingness to voice sensitive, revealing details about your life—hopes, disappointments, struggles, tragedies, humiliations, secrets—would inspire and depend on my willingness to do the same, and we'd each expect the other to receive such information with interest, acceptance, and a supportive attitude. We'd also expect each other to graciously receive any concerns or criticisms that either of us thought appropriate to voice—we'd welcome or at least tolerate the other holding us to account. Such a commitment to open-hearted sharing would strengthen a sense of our being an "us," which would, in turn, contribute to our being indifferent to our differences. This is a fine template for friendship but not for professional relationships. R. Epstein (2017) detailed how and why it goes wrong.

> If I assume that what I am feeling is exactly what the patient is feeling, I would be wrong much of the time. I've made the mistake of mentioning to patients who've had kidney stones that I've had them too. Some patients take this as an empathic gesture,[1] which leads to a sense of shared experience, but more often my self-disclosure falls flat; patients want me to understand *their* unique experience. They're interested in *their* kidney stones and aren't particularly interested in mine. Although I might think I understand their pain, their bland responses to my revelation confirm that I'm off the mark. (p. 130, italic in original)

At the end of the session with Jeanine and Cody, Randall rejoined the team behind the mirror. He told us he'd been taken aback by Cody's rude behavior. It felt, he said, a little like a slap in the face and that he'd have to think twice before "putting . . . [himself] out there" like that again. His reaction was no doubt complicated and intensified by the fact that the exchange with Cody had been "on display," witnessed by me and his five colleagues from behind the mirror. I mused aloud that it must have been disconcerting to have his well-intentioned sharing ignored and his reassurance of understanding dismissed. He nodded. We talked about that for a while, and then I offered an alternative approach to initiating empathic connections that wouldn't leave him feeling exposed and overextended and wouldn't leave his clients feeling misunderstood and disrespected. This book is an elaboration of that conversation.

What I didn't point out at the time (because I didn't yet know how to recognize and thus articulate it) was that Randall's interpretation of Cody's behavior as rude was predicated on an implicit expectation of symmetrical reciprocity ("If I'm respectful of you, you should respond in kind") and mutuality ("Your willingness to be open and vulnerable with me should match my willingness to be similarly open and vulnerable with you"). Such expectations have the potential to complicate and even undermine therapeutic relationships. For example, clients who like their therapists and see them as peers may attempt to initiate a friendship or romantic liaison.

---

[1] In my terms, the gesture would be an instance of analogy-inflected empathy (see p. 57, this volume).

My wife, Shelley, who is also a therapist, once saw a woman client about her age who suggested that they start holding their sessions at the wine bar across the street from our private practice. Supportive of the warm-hearted spirit of her client's idea, Shelley nevertheless clarified why it couldn't and wouldn't happen.

The young women therapists in the student counseling clinic I directed were regularly put in similar, though more challenging, positions. They sometimes talked in group supervision about how their male clients were constantly hitting on them. Such requests were understandable—why wouldn't a person who felt deeply heard and respected want to extend the experience of professional intimacy beyond the confines of the office? But to ensure that the relationships stayed therapeutic, the therapists, like my wife, needed to politely and clearly decline their clients' offers.

More problematic and ethically fraught are exchanges in which the clinician introduces a quality of mutuality into the professional relationship. Clients have mentioned during intake sessions with me that over the course of their working with their previous therapist, they ended up feeling like they, themselves, had become the professional. Even though they had continued paying for their sessions, the nature of the conversations had gradually shifted over time. Early on, the focus had been on their concerns, but toward the end, they found themselves addressing mostly the problems of the therapist. They'd felt special when their therapist first started revealing intimate details about personal struggles and/or frustrations with other clients, but at some point, they'd begun to feel taken advantage of, burdened by the responsibilities of listening and offering solace.

And then there are the clinicians who get sexually involved with a client. A year after a psychoanalyst, Sergio, started having sex with one of his female patients, he broke off the relationship and called me for an appointment. With deep shame and confusion, he said he wanted to sort out how, after a 20-year career in which he faithfully adhered to his profession's ethical code, he had, as he described it, "crossed a line." He said during his first appointment that only by making sense of what had gone wrong could he hope to trust himself not to cross it again.

Sergio said he'd seen this particular patient for a couple of years without anything untoward passing between them. But then, one day, at the end of an emotional session, the patient, "feeling raw," requested a "reassuring hug," and he, thinking nothing of it, provided it. At the end of the next two appointments, the same exchange unfolded. This seemed to enshrine a now-expected session-closing embrace. Before long, he was not just willingly participating in their "little ritual"; he had started looking forward to it. He'd been dealing with loneliness and various disappointments in his personal life, so the physicality of the hugs proved reassuring and pleasant. At some point down what he considered a slippery slope from professional to personal intimacy, their embraces lengthened and changed in meaning. The gestalt shift was marked by an impassioned kiss, which heralded the beginning of an intense affair. Sergio immediately fired himself as his new lover's therapist, but it took him many months to begin considering and then acknowledging the professional and personal ramifications of the path he'd taken.

I questioned Sergio's assumption that therapeutic and sexual intimacy lie along a tilted continuum, a slope that puts you in ever-present danger, if you're not treading carefully, of slip-sliding your way into the waiting arms of a desirable or desiring patient. Nonexploitive, intimate sexual relationships are characterized by a commitment to mutuality; they involve shared caring and pleasuring and, even more intensely than in friendships, shared vulnerability. But as with empathy, the relational shape of a nonexploitive therapeutic relationship is characterized by a commitment to asymmetrical complementarity. Such a stance is illustrated in Carl Rogers's (1989b) gentle but clear response to a client who desperately wanted to have sex with him. He told her, "The answer would be no. . . . I would not be willing to do that" (Rogers, 1989b, p. 131).

Sergio's identity as a therapist shifted—okay, crashed and burned—long before he became aroused or before the first kiss was exchanged. He didn't glide along a continuum; he took a sideways step from one relational universe into another, and it happened the moment he found himself enjoying or feeling grateful for his patient's embrace and looking forward to the next one.

Empathic and, more broadly, therapeutic, intimacy is safe so long as the client's despair, stories, openness, and requests for help or sex are not met with a reciprocal or analogous feeling or signaling of sympathetic vulnerability or need. Expressions of desired, imagined, or actual mutuality are warning signs that your commitment to dovetail complementarity is in jeopardy.

Had Sergio called me or a supervisor the moment he found himself wanting something gratifying from his patient, he could have taken steps to preempt his calamitous choice—referring his client to another therapist before his desire and arousal resulted in his reaching out to her. But also, more fundamentally, he'd have been able to safely probe his understanding of what constitutes a therapeutic relationship and overhaul his concomitant expectations of himself and his client(s). This, unfortunately, came after, not before, the harm was done.

Sergio's sexual transgression with his patient was miles removed from Randall's empathy blunder with Cody. However, each therapist failed to protect the inherent dovetail complementarity of professional intimacy, instead approaching the relationship with their client as an occasion for mutual, personal intimacy. Rather than reaching out with a self-focused need—to be recognized and appreciated, say, as a wounded healer (Randall) or as a desirable lover (Sergio)—the therapists were being called on, as are all clinicians, to engage with self-less care, committed to being fully present and respecting the integrity of the client's experience and boundaries.

EMBRACING IGNORANCE

不　知
知　不
知　知
病　上

Knowing ignorance: tiptop[2]
Ignorant knowing: defective
—Lao Tzu, in Douglas Flemons's *Completing Distinctions* (1991, p. 88)

If, like Randall, you've gone through something that lives in the same experiential zip code as a circumstance or condition your client is facing, you too might assume that your personal history grants you an automatic backstage pass to their inner world and gives you the requisite authority to work with them. And, as long as your client isn't a newly grieving 11-year-old boy named Cody and you don't try to shove what you know down the person's throat (more on that later), they might well prefer you to be their therapist, precisely because your and their life experiences rhyme in a meaningful way. You can earn street cred by having once floundered in the same hell in which they currently find themselves. You made it out alive, so it's possible they'll consider you perfectly positioned to now turn around and lend a helping hand. However, the idea that your personal story grants you automatic expertise on the experience of others is, in fact, a problematic assumption, one that gets in the way of your developing and communicating an empathic understanding of your client's unique challenges and resources.

> People often mistakenly believe that . . . [self-oriented perspective taking] provides them with access to the other's point of view when it does not. Most of us have had the experience of disclosing something to a friend, having her respond, "I know just how you are feeling," and then realizing within moments that she does not. It is not that she has not been perspective taking; she has. But the perspective has been *her own*—only the circumstances are ours. Thus, our friend's perspective taking has focused on her, not on us. While this can be useful for many reasons, it does not yield empathy. [We assume] that we "get" the other's experience when actually we do not. (Coplan, 2011b, p. 56, italic in original)

You perhaps know people who use the word *ignorant* as a synonym for *stupid*. They aren't stupid for doing so, but they *are* ignorant of the word's

---
[2]Chinese characters are read top to bottom and right to left.

Latin roots: The first letter comes from the Latin *in*, meaning "not," and *gnorant* comes from *gnōr-āre*, meaning "to know," so the word literally means "not to know." Not knowing something is, in and of itself, not generally a problem, particularly if you are aware of your ignorance. Indeed, Socrates's knowledge of his lack of knowledge was, he believed, the source of his wisdom, and known unknowns (Dunning, 2011) are the cornerstone of scientific discovery. According to Firestein (2012), good science critically depends on an embrace of ignorance, on the ability to discern when there is an "absence of fact, understanding, insight, or clarity about something" (p. 6). Grasping what we don't grasp, knowing what we don't know, is a form of "knowledgeable ignorance, perceptive ignorance, insightful ignorance," making it possible "to frame better questions, the first step to getting better answers" (Firestein, 2012, p. 6).

Dunning (2011) illuminated the ironic tangle that happens when we are both ignorant of something and ignorant of the fact of our ignorance: "People's ignorance is often invisible to them—... they suffer, for lack of a better term, a *meta-ignorance*, remaining ignorant of the multitude of ways they demonstrate gaps in knowledge" (p. 251). Unfortunately, but perhaps predictably, people's lack of such insight is often accompanied by their "firm sense that they are knowledgeable" (Dunning, 2011, p. 251). As Randall discovered, when your ignorance is sealed tight by certainty, impervious to feedback, empathy disappears. Cody's anger ignited into rage when Randall, doubly removed, doubly out of it, warmly dismissed Cody's assertion that he, Randall, didn't understand him: "No, really, I actually *do* [understand]," he said, "I went through it myself, so I totally get it." Smugly held meta-ignorance is infuriating.

One day, in a prepracticum course in my master's program, I was assigned the role of "counselor" and asked to practice active listening skills with my assigned "client," a short female classmate probably 10 years my senior. The whole exchange felt awkward. I stumbled over cheesy-sounding stock phrases (e.g., "What I hear you saying is . . ."; "It sounds like you're saying . . ."; "If I'm hearing you correctly, . . ."), but also, it seemed like whatever I said was bouncing off some unexplained chip on my partner's shoulder. I later relayed this piercingly perceptive observation to my professor, Dianne, who met with us one-on-one to go over the video recording of each week's practice session. Fortunately for me, she helped me locate and peer into my ignorance.

"How tall are you?" she asked.

"Six-two."

"Right. Going through life, seeing the world from that height, seeing it through your male eyes, you might not recognize how you come across to a woman who is more than a foot shorter than you. Even when you're both sitting down, she's looking up at you. You take up a lot of space in the room, your voice is deep, your face is serious, and you're used to being listened to just because of who and what you are. Are you aware that you can intimidate other people without even trying? You were thinking she had a chip on her shoulder? Got any other ideas?"

Dianne's wake-up call sparked a memory, which I relayed. A few years earlier, heading home alone on a cold, dark winter night, I was lost in thought as I walked quickly along what I assumed was a deserted street. Except it wasn't. Without realizing it, my pace had brought me up fast and close behind a woman walking less hurriedly than I. Hearing my swift footfalls, she had startled and turned around. I saw fear in her eyes, and, recognizing instantly that nothing I said, no matter how reassuring, could alter the fact that I'd scared her, I kept my mouth shut and immediately crossed the road.

The luxury of being able to safely walk alone at night, not feeling the need to monitor my surroundings because I wasn't worried about getting mugged or raped, is an excellent illustration of my White, tall, straight male privilege. Such "social patterns of not noticing, or inattention, are . . . the essence of cultural blind spots" (A. Friedman, 2019, p. 471), a "feature of cultural privilege" (p. 472). As Maibom (2022) pointed out,

> People who belong to the majority group, whose vision of life and well-being is culturally sanctioned and promoted in social policy, popular culture, and the arts, find it easy to ignore that *their* vision of life, of other people, and the world is *a* vision. (p. 223, italic in original)

The meta-ignorance of privilege-maintained blind spots can significantly limit our ability even to recognize, never mind grasp, the precarious realities of clients who are members of oppressed communities (see Elliott et al., 2018). Our knowing is limited by the perceptual fact that whatever we're able to take for granted becomes an assumed truth, an unquestioned foundation for our everyday experience. Those of us in privileged positions are freed from needing to consider or monitor the status of various elements and conditions relevant to our well-being unless and until we perceive them to be under threat—clean air and water, affordable food, reliable electricity, and safe, affordable housing and transportation; democracy, free speech, human rights, secure borders, and honored trade, peace, and arms agreements; and respected racial, cultural, sexual, and gender identities. Wittgenstein (1953) underscored that

> the aspects of things that are most important for us are hidden because of their simplicity and familiarity. (One is unable to notice something—because it is always before one's eyes). . . . And this means: we fail to be struck by what, once seen, is most striking and most powerful. (p. 50e)

According to Pedersen et al. (2008), "Privilege is not only a state of being preferred or favored but also a set of conditions that systematically empower select groups . . . while systematically not empowering others" (p. 82). In exchanges with clients from marginalized communities, we face limits to our seeing and understanding but also our saying. Flaskas (2018) described "the contextual colonial relations" in Australia, where she, "an otherwise sensible and nice white family therapist," was unable, as she put it, to "find an emotional place within myself to know how to speak of pain and sorrow with Aboriginal people without feeling as if I was (or am still) inflicting this pain, and so this knowing was banished from 'my agenda'" (p. 56). She noted that such "cultural not-knowingness . . . [can be] dangerous" (Flaskas, 2018, p. 62), particularly "where there is a living history of oppression" (p. 61).

Dianne continued helping me render my ignorance less meta: "And in the next week or two, you'll be doing a practice session with Devi (an Indian Canadian classmate), who is at risk, every day, of being demeaned and threatened by people who look like you and me. She can't not stay alert to the possibility of that. You can't do much to alter your appearance or your identity, but you can be ready for her alertness, perhaps her wariness. And respect it—the legitimacy of it. That will be difficult if you're interpreting it as a chip on her shoulder."

This was the first time I'd been systematically invited to recognize and probe a cultural blind spot and my concomitant biases. I found it humbling and unsettling but also intriguing. I didn't realize it at the time, but Dianne's challenge opened the door to empathy, wonder, and curiosity about the other.

As Pedersen et al. (2008) pointed out, "those of us who have different forms of privilege commonly have a great deal of difficulty acknowledging" it (p. 82). I've been fortunate that in the 40 years since my class with Dianne, my wife, daughter, son, students, colleagues, friends, and some intrepid clients (mostly teenagers) have each, on occasion, taken it upon themselves to point out times when I've failed to see and/or understand that I was failing to see and/or understand. Clearly, identifying meta-ignorance isn't a one-and-done undertaking. Flaskas (2018) advised staying ever observant and ever curious:

> I am inclined to think that the . . . [most] important question in terms of my practice and politics is . . . "what can I know?" What, in my particular context, with this particular family, are the limits and capacities of my knowing and understanding? And how can I stay alert to the power of my limits while nurturing my capacities to attempt to know and understand the interplay of difference and sameness in . . . all my psychotherapy work? (pp. 67–68)

One way to stay alert to your ignorance of your ignorance is to welcome and learn from any illuminating feedback, whether requested or not, offered up by people in your personal and professional worlds.

NOT PRESUMING

Empathy requires knowing you know nothing.
—Leslie Jamison, *The Empathy Exams* (2014)

I think . . . of the remark Derrida is reputed to have made some years ago when asked where his thought was headed: "I am trying precisely to put myself at a point so that I do not know any longer where I am going."
—Jerome A. Miller, *Wonder As Hinge* (1989, p. 53)

What we experience as "certainty"—the feeling of knowing what is true about ourselves, each other, and the world around us—is an illusion that the brain manufactures to help us make it through each day. Giving up a bit of that certainty now and then is a good idea.
—Lisa Feldman Barrett, *How Emotions Are Made* (2017a, p. 288)

My friend Gabe once described to me how frustrating it was to divulge any life difficulty to her now-deceased older sister. The sister would "co-opt . . . [other people's problems] if they resonated even vaguely" with something she had faced, rushing to assert, "It happened to me too, only worse." Gabe said, "She . . . [told] me once that a relationship struggle I was having in my forties was something she'd gone through herself . . . in her teens" (M. Hesthammar, personal communication, July 11, 2022).

Certainty withers curiosity (cf. Cecchin, 1987, pp. 409–410). If your client's current struggles remind you of something you faced and dealt with in the past, then, like Randall or Gabe's sister, you may be certain that you already know what it is like to be them. However, if your client's current struggles remind you of something you never resolved and/or are still dealing with in the present, then you may be certain that you have nothing to offer them. In this instance, instead of prompting hubris, your certainty invites self-doubt or self-recrimination. In either case, empathy—and the therapeutic relationship—takes a hit. I've seen more than one client over the years who was failing to stay sober while working as a therapist in a recovery setting. They were sure they were nothing but useless frauds. And with much of their focus consumed by not getting outed, the bandwidth necessary for being fully present for and curious about their patients was severely attenuated.

I remember once supervising an intern, Lissette, who wondered if she should transfer a new client who had come to the first session requesting help for a crippling fear of heights. As someone who, herself, couldn't go near gondolas, rooftop bars, or apartment balconies, Lissette was afraid that she was the worst possible person to be his therapist. She fretted whether she should be honest and tell him about her own struggles, but she feared that if she "came clean," it would undermine his respect for her and would further convince him that his problem was hopeless. The onslaught of questions she posed to herself had kept her from finding many—indeed, any—useful details about her client's experience.

I suggested that the idea of Lissette's "owing it" to her client to be "genuine" was grounded in the misplaced conception that her fear of heights existed inside her as an isolable entity, stripped of the context of her personal history and relationships. Viewing it this way resulted in her considering her fear to be the same as, and thus directly relevant to, her client's. As we talked, she allowed for the fact that their respective difficulties with heights were distinct in more than just degree of severity; they also differed in how and in what circumstances they cropped up.

I agreed with Lissette that "confessing" to the client her history of grappling with heights would unhelpfully change her relationship with him. Offering up her history of distress would undermine the complementarity of her empathically making sense of—and exploring possibilities for change in—her client's experience. Instead, she would be inviting a symmetry-shaped interaction, with each of them sympathetically commiserating with the other regarding their shared affliction. If Lissette and her client were friends, then revealing her history of distress would no doubt contribute to their growing closer and more mutually trusting; however, given that she was her client's therapist, her job was to self-lessly delve into his story without presuming any privileged grasp of his challenges and possibilities. As H. Anderson and Goolishian (1992) put it,

> Therapists are always prejudiced by their experience, but . . . they must listen in such a way that their pre-experience does not close them to the full meaning of the client's descriptions of their experience. This can only happen if the therapist approaches each clinical experience from the position of not knowing. To do otherwise is to search for regularities and common meaning that may validate the therapist's theory but invalidate the uniqueness of the clients' stories and thus their very identity. (p. 30)

Shunryu Suzuki (2006) advised that "when you listen to someone, you should give up all your preconceived ideas and your subjective opinions" (p. 102). Certainty gums up your ability to truly listen and be fully present (Geller & Greenberg, 2023). The alternative is to encounter the client with, as phenomenology researchers would say, your biases bracketed (Chan et al., 2013) or with what Suzuki (2006) called "beginner's mind," emptied of self-centered thoughts. "A mind full of preconceived ideas, subjective intentions, or habits is not open to things as they are. That is why we practice zazen [i.e., sitting meditation]: to clear our mind of what is related to something else" (Suzuki, 2006, p. 104).

Hirshfield confirmed Suzuki's notion of beginner's mind as a form of meditative awareness: "You are always hoping to be inside whatever moment it is you find yourself . . . as if it were new to you, as if you didn't know what it is" (Shaheen, 2023, 31:45). The novelist George Saunders said that the goal for him while writing is to "get to the place where your usual judging mind has been quieted. . . . All your usual easy opinions just get reduced, and you're just in that holy state of not knowing anything, which is a kind of sacred place, really" (Colbert, 2022, 04:02). You want to be able to draw from your experience and expertise with neither it nor your certainty about it getting in your way:

> Suzuki Roshi said, "Not-knowing does not mean you don't know." It doesn't require us to forget everything we have known or to suspend all interpretations of a situation. Not-knowing means not being limited by what we know, holding what we know lightly so that we are ready for it to be different. Maybe things are this way. But maybe they are not. (Fronsdal, 2003, 22:25)

There's no way of getting around the fact that your personal history and professional expertise, experience, and responsibilities will come into play in some way or other during therapeutic encounters (Laird, 2000). You'd be negligent if you disregarded them as sources of guidance; however, if you place them as filters *between* you and the client, you risk your conversations merely confirming what you already knew you knew rather than opening you to discovery, to learning about the client's uniqueness from inside the patterns and embodied logic of their world.

Earlier, I quoted Firestein (2012) saying that "insightful ignorance" makes it possible for scientists "to frame better questions, the first step to getting better answers" (p. 6). Good therapy similarly depends on wisely cultivating ignorance so we can meet each client each time with a fresh openness and availability to connect, learn, and discover. For us, framing better questions is the first step to opening possibilities for therapeutic change. Unfortunately, the notion of "not knowing" has been misunderstood by some as referring to therapists "lacking knowledge, feigning ignorance, withholding knowledge, avoiding suggestions, or forgetting what . . . [they] know" (H. Anderson, 2001, p. 350). To avoid such confusion, I prefer to talk about empathy as a commitment to not presuming—a way of organizing and arraying the details of your personal history and professional expertise not *between* you and the client but *behind* you, in the background of your awareness.

The uncluttered simplicity of not presuming to know clears the way for unencumbered projective imagining, which is central to both writing fiction

(Saunders, as cited in Fragoso, 2023) and engaging empathically. As Halpern (2001) put it, "Curiosity requires suspending judgment and allowing oneself to be uncertain. As such, it directs empathy toward ongoing discovery" (p. 130). Like an improv performer, you prepare assiduously to initiate and respond with contextually sensitive spontaneity, trusting yourself, the other, and the process (J. Gale, personal communication, August 19, 2024). If you proceed tentatively, feeling your way, step by step, your client can discover "what a relief it is to be in the company of someone confident enough to stay unsure (that is, perpetually curious)" (Saunders, 2021, p. 338).

Not presuming involves treating relevant details of your life history as sources of color in the palette of your imagination, indirectly helping you choose descriptors and articulate floated hunches (see Chapter 5) as you empathically launch your self-less curiosity across the self–other divide. Instead of searching your memory for an analog of the other's circumstance so that you can relate to their experience, you're much better off leaving *your* self and *your* history out of the equation so you can imaginatively conjure the *client's* embodiment in the *client's* story (see Truax & Carkhuff, 1967, p. 288).

In 2017, the singer-songwriter Ed Sheeran was sued for copyright infringement of Marvin Gaye and Ed Townsend's song "Let's Get It On" (Seabrook, 2023). Lawyers for the plaintiff, Ed Townsend's daughter, claimed that "the melodic, harmonic, and rhythmic compositions" of Sheeran's song "Thinking Out Loud" were "substantially and/or strikingly similar" to "Let's Get It On" (Seabrook, 2023, para. 37). The case went to trial in 2023, and, as part of his defense, Sheeran, pulling out his guitar in the courtroom, documented and demonstrated that almost all pop songs share similar chord progressions and structural features: "You can kind of play most pop songs over most pop songs" (Seabrook, 2023, para. 70) he testified. Nevertheless, while employing these common characteristics, musicians are able to create remarkably distinctive tunes, each with its own identifying fingerprints, its own idiosyncratic rhythmic, melodic, harmonic, and lyrical integrity.[3]

As with music, so with people. You wouldn't have the ability to form impressions of your clients empathically, outlined and saturated with the details being relayed in your conversations with them, if it weren't for the fact that you, like them, have lived a life peppered with hope and despair, trust and betrayal, pleasure and pain, desire and disgust, support and abandonment, achievements and failures, curiosity and fear, reassurance and uncertainty. Your experience displays intra- and interpersonal patterns common across

---

[3] Sheeran won the case; the jury decided that regardless of shared features between the two tunes, he had independently composed "Thinking Out Loud."

human relating. But when you begin homing in on and teasing out textures and nuanced shapes, as well as sources of light and shadow, that are unique to the other person's story, any thoughts about or focus on the specifics of your personal journey are irrelevant to and a distraction from coming to know, presumption-free, the signature particularities of the other.

NOT JUDGING

The highest expression of empathy is accepting and nonjudgmental.
—Carl R. Rogers, *Empathic* (1975, p. 7)

Many people believe the way to be nonjudgmental is to be more accepting of others and to accept their "weaknesses." My view is quite different. I believe that recognizing the sense to someone else's behavior is a path to being nonjudgmental.
—Ellen Langer, *The Mindful Body* (2023)

As I explained in Chapter 1, judgment inscribes a self–other boundary, setting you apart from whatever or whomever you are evaluating. When the judgment is negative, it puts you at odds, or even in contention with, whatever you're considering unacceptable, alien. But even a positive appraisal inscribes a boundary between your sense of self and the experience "you" are having. Jay Haley (1981, p. 241) told a story of a Zen teacher's response to a student who gushed, "Isn't the mountain beautiful?" The teacher replied, "Yes, but isn't it a pity to say so?" This is why mindfulness meditation traditions advise you to attune your awareness toward a simple acknowledgment of the fact of what's happening without putting an evaluative stamp on it.

The boundary imposed through negative judgment keeps your sense of self—along with your values and beliefs—safe from being disarrayed, contaminated, or undermined by whatever or whomever you deem other or alien. However, in constituting and sustaining your disapproval, your judgment precludes meaningful connection or empathic understanding. I know this firsthand. My wife, Shelley, and I (along with 25 other people) once missed a late-evening connection in the Charlotte airport because of a delayed departure from Palm Springs caused by a problem with the plane's air-conditioning. We would need to stay the night, but the airline's customer service agent said she couldn't issue us a hotel voucher because, according to the information on her computer, the delay had been caused by inclement weather. At my request, the agent called over her supervisor, Ron, and we had the following conversation. I was already steamed.

RON: I just talked with air traffic control in Palm Springs, and they confirmed that the flight departed on time. We don't provide hotel or taxi vouchers for weather delays.

DOUGLAS: But it wasn't a weather delay. It's true that we left the gate on time, but we then sat on the tarmac for an hour. Planes were leaving all around us. The AC wasn't working—water was dripping on passengers' heads. The pilot announced over the intercom that a mechanic had come out from the hangar to work on it.

Ron then doubled down, and I matched him. Remember my talking earlier about symmetrical interactions? This was a good example of one involving the sympathetic resonance of judgment-infused irritation.

RON: Both our records and air traffic control confirm that it was a weather delay.

DOUGLAS: Except it wasn't. The information in your system is not accurate.

We each had our backs up in response to the other—in response to someone we each viewed as alien. I wish I could tell you that my getting caught in this escalation took place a long time ago, but, in fact, it happened recently—I'd already started working on this book.

RON: You keep repeating yourself.

I have no idea how long we would have continued hopelessly spiraling if another passenger standing just behind me, Ken, hadn't stepped in.

KEN: So, Ron, your system shows that we were late because of a weather delay. You went to the trouble to call traffic control in Palm Springs, and they confirmed that.

Finally, someone capable of empathy! Ken had just joined us, and he'd already ventured inside Ron's version of the situation.

RON: That's correct.

KEN: So I guess your hands are tied. You have no way of issuing us vouchers unless the system shows a mechanical problem, and it doesn't say that. You have to rely on what the system tells you.

RON: Exactly. I will talk only with you, because you are being reasonable.

He was exactly right. I was too tired and incensed (read judgmental) to be reasonable. Nevertheless, I could recognize and be impressed (and somewhat chagrined) by Ken's skillful empathic engagement.

KEN: And they haven't given you the authority to override what it says in the computer.

RON: They have not.

Note that Ken was implying that Ron would have helped us if he'd only had the authority to do so. I'm not sure this indirect attribution of positive intent was true, but it helped to ease Ron out of his role and identity as the enemy. Ken also managed to subtly underscore, without blame, that the information in the computer was faulty.

KEN: That's gotta be frustrating. You have to answer to a bunch of irate, stranded passengers, but the airline doesn't give you the tools necessary to find a resolution.

Brilliant. Ken was joining with Ron over how hard it must be, this late at night, to have his hands tied when having to deal with the likes of me.

In response to Ken's comments, Ron's tone changed dramatically.

RON: There's nothing I can do, I'm afraid.

KEN: Yeah, I get that. And there's probably no one here at this hour who could.

There wasn't a hint of snark in Ken's statement, and Ron could tell. When freed from having to defend himself, Ron could clearly lay out our available (albeit not ideal) options.

RON: No. You can stay in the airport tonight if you want to. If you go to a hotel, you'll have to pay for it yourself, but tomorrow you can file a report.

As we stranded passengers all got ready to go our separate ways, I turned to Ken, thanked him for his adroit handling of the situation, and asked him about his professional background. He told me he was an audiologist who dealt with clients and employees "every day, all day long."[4] Unlike me, he'd been able to bring his work skills online right when they were needed, despite the late

---

[4] I also got his contact information. Anticipating that the exchange would be an excellent illustration for this book, I wanted to be able to confirm with him that my account of the dialogue (which I ended up scribbling down in the taxi on the way to our hotel) aligned with what he recalled.

hour and the challenge of dealing with an intransigent, officious bureaucrat (see, there I go again).

In the course of your career, you may occasionally find judgment similarly standing in the way of your joining with a client, preventing your empathic imagination from self-lessly crossing the self–other border. This happened to me when, as a doctoral student, I was asked to see a man who had just walked into our training clinic, asking for an immediate appointment (I first talked about this case in *Of One Mind*; Flemons, 2002, pp. 44–45). For the next 50 minutes, he never took off his mirrored sunglasses.

The man told me that earlier that day, his wife had once again taken the kids and walked out, insisting that she wouldn't return until he'd gone to therapy. So, even though he wasn't happy about it, he was doing what she'd demanded so he could get her to come back. He was willing to jump through whatever hoops necessary, but he didn't know yet how many sessions it would take to do the trick. Once he found out, he'd book the lot of them, maybe one a day, so he could get them all done as quickly as possible. What he did know, he said, was that when she got back, he'd be slapping some sense into her. Where did she get off telling *him* what *he* had to do? This wasn't the first time she'd up and left, but he assured me it would be her last. Next time, he and his gun would be voicing an opinion.

The man's cold rage scared the hell out of me. I was terrified for the safety of his family but, concerned that he might have brought a concealed weapon to the appointment, also my own. Too unnerved to empathize, I kept him at arm's length and told him I had a problem. "If I see you for therapy," I said, "and you tell your wife about it, she may decide it is worth it to try again with you. But then, if she does come back, she's going to get beat up. And then, if the therapy is good enough to get her to return to you but not good enough to keep her from walking out again, she'll be in danger of getting shot. That's too big a risk for me. I don't want to be a part of someone dying."

He leaned toward me and whispered, "Don't worry; no one will ever know I was here. I won't tell nobody. Not even the cops. They'll never get it out of me." I thanked him for his vow of silence but stuck to my decision. I should have offered him names and numbers of other clinics or therapists he could try, but I have no memory of doing so. After he left, I contacted a colleague at the local Women in Distress to see if they could pass along a safety alert.

Because my fear-induced judgment never abated, my seeing him as alien never wavered. I was able to transport my imagination inside his wife's story, but because I hadn't yet figured out that both–and empathizing is possible (see Chapter 5), I couldn't enter his. I left him in the lurch.

Years later, one of the students in a clinical practicum I was supervising, Irma, experienced a similar recoiling from someone she deemed too alien to work with. Irma was on deck to take the next case assigned to our team: a former crack addict, Mick, in recovery for 2 years, who wanted help stopping what had become a compulsive behavior—torturing his mother's cats when she wasn't home (for an elaborated discussion of the case, see Flemons, 2002, pp. 51, 52, 58–68). Irma, an animal activist who worked tirelessly on behalf of homeless cats in Miami, coordinated a spay and neuter program and lobbied for stiffer penalties for animal abusers. She considered herself exactly the wrong person to be Mick's therapist. Rather than assign the case to another student, I decided to see Mick myself, which allowed Irma to observe with the rest of the team from behind the one-way mirror. Even this proved challenging for her; watching our conversations, she often felt physically ill.

Mick told me in the first session that when he was at work, he would get a rush, almost as if he were high, as he imagined what he would do to the cats when he got home. In the second session, he revealed that he had, a few weeks earlier, killed one of the cats. This news outraged and horrified Irma, who considered him a monster, a sadist.

And me? If I hadn't been Mick's therapist and if, say, I'd been out for a walk and had witnessed his abusing his mother's pets through a window, I would have been as sickened and outraged as Irma. I would have immediately called the police to report him, and like Irma, I'd have endorsed his receiving a stiff sentence. But given confidentiality and my ethical obligations as a therapist, a different response was called for. Relating to him as an alien or enemy, dismissively recoiling from him, was not an option. Instead, I projected my untethered imagination into the heart of his story—into his sensations, perceptions, fears, urges, choices, despair, and relationships. In the process, my sense of self became temporarily irrelevant as the horrific logic of hurting the cats holographically emerged as a graspable sensibility.

Ralph Fiennes played Lord Voldemort in the Harry Potter films, and some years earlier, in *Schindler's List*, he portrayed the SS officer Amon Goeth. Fiennes considers acting "above all an exercise in imagination" (Hirschberg, 2006, para. 5). An otherwise decent person (Maibom, 2022, p. 241), he is, according to a New York theater director, "good at monsters.... He doesn't approach them sensationally. He tries to understand them" (Dowd, 2022, para. 10). Fiennes imagines the person he is playing "from the inside out" (Hirschberg, 2006, para. 5) from "the gut to the heart to the head" (para. 3). For him, "so much of movie acting is in loving your characters. I try to know them, and with that intimacy comes love.... I love Voldemort" (Hirschberg, 2006, para. 6).

Love is unencumbered acceptance, a constellation of care, understanding, and appreciation toward which Carl Rogers (1980) gestured with his notion of the "non-possessive prizing" of "unconditional positive regard" (p. 116).

Nonjudgment is an essential ingredient of such engagement, and love is an appropriate characterization of the intimacy of the unbounded nature of such relationships. Nevertheless, I wouldn't say that, in the spirit of Ralph Fiennes, I loved Mick. As I detailed in Chapter 2, empathic engagement involves checking your circumscribed self at the door, so my "I" is out of the picture when I'm self-lessly projecting my imagination into the sense and story of the other's experience. There is a quality of love in the enterprise, but "I" am not feeling it. It is held in the relationship.

I can tell I'm empathically locked in when the client reveals something that a nontherapist would find unnerving, and my immediate response is not, "Wait, what? No! You did what?! How could you?!" Rather, I'm registering, from inside, the logic and embodied position of the client and thus, without my eyebrows raised or my guard up, "Yes, of course! That fits exactly. That makes sense." The client's otherness dissipates with your judgment when you project your imagination across the self–other divide and make inside sense of the person's experience within the context, the web, of the intra- and interpersonal relationships weaving their story. If there's any othering going on, it will be found in the client's critical self-assessment. Communicating an empathic understanding of this judgmental attitude won't drive a wedge between you and the client; it will forge greater trust (Lopez, 1987). This can be clearly seen in the work of the psychiatrist and clinical hypnosis pioneer Milton Erickson.

Carl Rogers and Milton Erickson each acknowledged commonalities between their two approaches (Erickson & Rossi, 2014, p. 51; Gunnison, 1985, p. 562; Rogers, 1987, p. 182); however, whereas Rogers (2007) considered empathy "a gentle way of being" (p. 3) involving nonpossessive warmth (Truax & Lister, 1970, p. 229), Erickson would sometimes speak with his patients in ways that, from the perspective of an outside observer, would have sounded harsh, cold, and distinctly critical (e.g., Erickson, 2008b, p. 75). According to Zeig, Erickson would establish "a high degree of empathic rapport" with his patients, but he did so implicitly (Erickson & Zeig, 2008, p. 286).

Erickson's patients heard what he was saying as an accurate reflection of their sense of self and their circumstances (Lopez, 1987). For example, he once worked with an obese young woman whose family members had all died. She believed that she, too, was destined to die soon, and she was certain that because of her appearance, Erickson would refuse to work with her. Erickson (2008b) concluded

> that the only possible understanding this girl had of intercommunication was that of unkindness and brutality. Hence, brutality would be used to convince her of [my] sincerity. Any other possible approach, any kindness, would be misinterpreted. She could not possibly believe courteous language. I realized that

rapport would have to be established—and established very quickly. She would have to be convinced, beyond a doubt, that I understood and recognized her and her problem and was not afraid to speak openly, freely, unemotionally, but truthfully. (p. 75)

Erickson delivered his "brutal truth" in the form of stinging criticisms of the client's appearance. This established a ground of agreement and trust between them that he subsequently built on to help her alter her relationship to herself and other people. Years later, when she was happily married with two adolescent children, the client said to Erickson (2008b), "When you said those awful things about me, you were so truthful. I knew that you were telling me the truth, that I could trust you. I am so glad you told me the truth" (p. 79). The intensity, attitude, and manner of speaking that Erickson adopted when conversing with his client was familiar territory for her and was the empathic foundation of the hypnotic work they did together.[5] Haley (1981) considered such a manner of relating deeply respectful:

> If a therapist is warm and empathic with a patient who is a cold fish, there is something wrong with that therapist and he should be more considerate. To be cold in that situation would be more appropriate and human. . . . The [patient] will feel that yet another person does not understand her. The therapist must join that [patient's] universe and from within that universe bring about change. (p. 239)

As I continued to work with Mick, he stopped, as he put it, "playing rugby" with the cats, and the urge to hurt them waned. He'd been attending Narcotics Anonymous meetings since stopping crack, but now, for the first time, he was actively participating in them, and he talked about going back to school. During the postsession team discussion after Mick's and my fifth or sixth appointment, I asked Irma if she could now be his therapist. "Yes," she said, "because today he said he didn't feel the urge to go after the cats. But if the urge were to come back, I don't think I could."

Of course, a commitment to empathy and therapeutic relationships in general can't be provisional. You need to either go all in or refer the case. Shapiro (2012) cautioned against the toe-dipping nature of *selective empathy*, which involves limiting your "emotional engagement and meaningful understanding" to "certain 'likeable' patients or patients similar to" (p. 280) you. When you undertake empathy as a "deeply held commitment to a way of being in the world," it can be "cultivated toward all patients, especially stigmatized, marginalized, or otherwise unappealing patient populations" (Shapiro, 2012, p. 280).

---

[5]This discussion of Erickson and his case originally appeared in Flemons (2022, pp. 64–65).

As I discussed in Chapter 3, you can and should manage your engagement so that you're able to freely move into and out of the self-less imagination required of empathic curiosity. In preparation for working with a client from whom you, as a regular person, would naturally recoil, you may need to take a few minutes to collect yourself and, perhaps as part of a mindfulness meditation ritual, acknowledge and accept each of your judgmental reactions as legitimate. They just don't need to accompany you into the session. There is room in your gym-style therapy locker at the back of your mind to store them, stacked neatly on the shelf beside your towel and your circumscribed self. You can always gather them back up at the end of the day if needed.

NOT CLAIMING

Show, don't tell.
–George Saunders, A Swim in a Pond in the Rain (2021)

Brené Brown (2018) suggested using phrases such as the following as an empathic means of connecting with those locked down by shame:

- Oh, man. I feel you.
- I know that feeling, and it sucks.
- Me too.
- I see you. You're not alone.
- I've been in a similar place, and it's really hard.
- I understand what that's like. (p. 160)

Each of these statements would be best characterized not as an expression of empathy but of empathy-inflected sympathy (see Chapter 1). They all reflect a commitment to the mutuality of sympathetic resonance and self-conscious awareness.

I had a warm, gregarious friend, Stuart, who, before he died, would have been perfectly capable of—and comfortable with—offering any of these assurances to someone in pain. He'd have meant what he said with every ounce of his generous being, and the recipient wouldn't have doubted for a second his good intentions. But would anyone have just taken his word on faith that he "got" them? I sure would have. We knew each other for a couple of decades, so he wouldn't have had to say much of anything for me to recognize the devoted and enveloping embrace of his attention. Any one of the statements would have served as a shorthand assertion of loving concern.

However, in relationships that don't have long-established, unquestioned care and trust stitched into the fabric of their being, such claims of understanding won't carry much weight. In my 30 years of hanging out behind one-way mirrors, watching sessions unfold in real time, I never saw a client simply accept and be moved by a therapist's declaration of empathic knowing. The client might not protest the therapist's avowal as directly or vociferously as Cody did Randall's, but absent a meaningful, preexisting connection to lend heft and heart to the therapists' assurances, the claims just didn't land.

I've also heard stories from clients about their failed, claim-based empathic efforts. Sean, a single dad, consulted with me about his "impossible" teenage son, Blake, who, diagnosed with depression, was struggling both in school and with friends. Blake consistently rebuffed Sean's efforts to ease some of his pain, shutting him out and shutting him down. Recently, Sean said Blake had come home and collapsed on the couch, griping about how horrible his day had been. Sean asked him what had happened, and Blake began telling him about these bullies a grade ahead of him who'd been making his life miserable, accosting him in the hallway and belittling him every chance they got. Soon into hearing what these older kids had done, Sean, in a sincere effort to connect, jumped in with what he assumed would be heard as enthusiastic empathic support. He only got as far as saying, "I know what that's like. When I was your age, I remember one time when . . .," before Blake blew up and stormed out of the room.

Do you know the creative writer's credo I cited in the epigraph to this section ("Show, don't tell")? It inspires authors to create more immersive, emotionally meaningful stories by sidestepping exposition in favor of descriptions of action and dialogue. "Rather than *asserting* something for the reader to *accept*, 'Show, don't tell' . . . *transmits* something for the reader to *experience*" (Glatch, 2022, "What Is 'Show, Don't Tell' Writing" section, italic in original). I propose an analogous clinician's credo: "Show, don't claim." Rather than presumptuously declaring possession of insider knowledge for the client to accept, "Show, don't claim" nonpresumptuously demonstrates an empathic grasp of the client's story for the client to recognize. Instead of asserting what you believe you already know, you sketch out what you're coming to understand (cf. Rogers & Farson, 1957/2021): "Empathy includes an appreciative feel for the story or narrative of a person or family, a capacity to resonate in various ways to the theme or themes involved and to articulate these appreciatively" (Perry, 1993, p. 70).

Sean was a loving dad who wanted to understand and help his son, and he wanted Blake to recognize his support. I suggested we role-play some replays of the ill-fated conversation about bullies and see where it might go. I started out playing Sean so that Sean, as Blake, could get a sense of what it is like to be on the receiving end of empathy being shown rather than claimed.

"SEAN": Tough day?

"BLAKE": You could say that.

"SEAN": The bullies?

"BLAKE": Yep.

"SEAN": Accosting you between classes or after school?

"BLAKE": Either. Both. Or at lunch.

"SEAN": Wherever, whenever—never quite sure.

"BLAKE": Yep. You never know.

"SEAN": So I guess no time, no place feels safe.

"BLAKE": Not really. Maybe in class.

"SEAN": But isn't it hard to concentrate, knowing the bell's going to ring and you'll be back out in the hallways?

"BLAKE": Sometimes.

"SEAN": Must be exhausting—needing to always be on the lookout, always on edge.

"BLAKE": You have no idea.

"SEAN": Nope, you're right. I don't.

Sean found the roleplay revelatory but objected to that last comment: "It's not accurate," he said. "I do know what it's like. Why say I don't?" The dad in him so wanted to rescue his son from the insularity of his suffering; he worried that if he were to acknowledge verbally the idea that he didn't know what his son was going through, then Blake would end up feeling more alone than he already did. We talked about how fundamental that worry was and the inevitable limits in knowing how anyone else processes their own experience, even if the circumstances they face are familiar to us. That made sense to him.

I then asked Sean what he had noticed during our dialogue. He said that besides the fact that he, as Blake, didn't get pissed off, he had also felt acknowledged. We agreed that this was a different way for a person not to feel alone. Rogers (1987) would have concurred. He said that "if a person can be *understood*, he or she *belongs*" (p. 181). Later, we switched it up so that Sean, playing himself, could get a feel, while dialoguing with me as Blake, for how to shift from certainty to curiosity and distill his memories of being bullied into wonderings and tentatively offered hunches about Blake's current hell.

I've often wondered how Randall's session with Cody could have unfolded differently if he'd been in a position to embrace and implement the ideas in this chapter. I will be offering a revised rendering of what unfolded that evening, but not yet. First, in the next (and final) chapter, I discuss and illustrate a variety of techniques of empathic engagement—skills that Randall would have found helpful for putting his reconsidered assumptions into practice.

5 SKILLS OF EMPATHIC ENGAGEMENT

Empathy is not a "thing" but a way of interacting.
—Anna Aragno, *The Language of Empathy* (2008, p. 714)

When we attune to others we allow our own internal state to shift, to come to resonate with the inner world of another. This resonance is at the heart of the important sense of "feeling felt" that emerges in close relationships.
—Daniel J. Siegel, *Mindsight* (2010)

A high degree of empathy in a relationship is possibly the *most potent factor in bringing about change and learning.*
—Carl R. Rogers, *A Way of Being* (1980, p. 139)

In Chapter 1, I told you a story about my family visiting a restaurant that offered the option of ordering "two soups in a bowl." The chef would simultaneously pour separate ladles of two differently colored (and flavored) thick soups into opposite sides of a bowl, each acting as a barrier to the unfettered spread of the other. As a result, as the bowl filled, a more-or-less straight line would form across the middle, where the two soups met. I asked the waiter for the two-soups option, but I requested that the chef pour the same soup from both ladles. When the waiter delivered the bowl to the table, it appeared to be filled with only one soup. With no contrast in color available to distinguish one side from the other, no boundary or line of demarcation could be detected by me or my family. The difference was indifferentiated.

A client offers an account of some circumstance they're facing, along with their response to it. And you, empathically engaged, project your self-less imagination into the heart of their story. As the narrative unfolds, you offer back distilled snippets of what they're describing. You mention what stands out to you, highlighting details of what happened, how the client felt about it, what they surmised, and/or what they chose to do.

Now, if you were to record the conversation and, listening back, juxtapose their telling and your retelling, you would notice that the more closely you hewed to what they said and how they said it, the more the two renditions would resemble a bowl of two side-by-side ladles of the same soup. They would be different, but the differences would be minimal. The usual metaphor for conveying this similarity is a mirror—the empathic therapist is said to "reflect" what the client is saying. As I discuss later, this depiction is problematic because it implies that there is one best empathic response—a description formulated for the client that precisely echoes their words and directly re-presents their emotional experience. A different conceptual metaphor is called for, one that properly acknowledges the important overlap—the redundancy—between the client's storytelling and the therapist's response but also takes into account the fact that emotions are constructed. In preparation for introducing and developing this metaphor, I need to illuminate some of the interpersonal, communicational dynamics of the empathic encounter. Let's start with redundancy.

THE BENEFITS OF REDUNDANCY

Consider the case in which I say to you, "It's raining," and you guess that if you look out the window you will see raindrops. . . . Few people in this situation restrain themselves from seemingly duplicating their information by looking out of the window. We like to prove that our guesses are right, and that our friends are honest. Still more important, we like to test or verify the correctness of our view of our relationship to others.
  —Gregory Bateson, *Steps to an Ecology of Mind* (1972/2000, pp. 141-142)

Redundancy is not an unfortunate by-product of empathic communication; it is, in some sense, the goal. It is sought. Which raises a question of relevance. What's the point? How does a client benefit from being offered a translated reiteration of their experience? I can point to three. First, when you show a client, rather than claim, that you understand something of their experience, they are provided evidence and assurance that they are not alone, that they are "no longer an isolate" (Rogers, 1975, p. 6). Accompaniment not only is essential as support for solo performers at music recitals but also is central to what it means to be a person. As the journalist Andy Crouch put it, "Recognition is the first human quest" (as cited in Brooks, 2023, p. 134), a truth reflected in the Latin roots of the word *conscious*: "to know" (*sci*) "together" (*con*). Whatever a baby's "first words actually seem to be saying," said Lewis Thomas (1990),

> the first urgent message—to parents, sisters and brothers, visitors, strangers on the sidewalk, the family dog—is "Think with me." And, once begun, this becomes life's mission for almost all of us. . . . "Think with me" is what we really mean when we use the term *consciousness*. When we say that we are conscious, we do not intend to say something important about the workings of own brains; we are talking, etymologically, about the minds of others. And this, of course, is what the language intended. Consciousness is knowing together. (pp. 114–115, italic in original)

Empathic communication demonstrates a felt consciousness, thinking-and-feeling *as* the other, derived from imagining and speaking your way into the knowing heart of their experience.

The second benefit of offering a faithful rendering of the client's experience has to do with your connection with the client. The better you're able to attune what you say and how you say it to accord with the content and expression of the client's story, the more the difference between the two renderings is diminished. This has the potential for the client to register your comments more as insider descriptions than as outsider evaluations (see Rogers, 1962, p. 419; 1989b, p. 128).

I remember a 16-year-old firecracker I saw who complained early on about how "sloooooooooowly" I spoke. Bright, funny, and impatient, she had no time for my measured comments. If I couldn't rattle off what I had to say, she wouldn't hear it because she was already onto something else. So as not to get left in the dust or kicked to the curb, I needed to up my game, or at least my pace, so I sped up the metronome in my larynx. A few weeks later, I mentioned in passing that she seemed less exasperated in our sessions. She shrugged her shoulders and allowed for the fact that I had become less annoying.

This fits with Maibom's (2022) observation that "the degree to which people are able to synchronize their natural rhythms seems to play a large role in their sense of connectedness. . . . A secret to smooth interactions with others is mutual entrainment of speech rhythms," which is "central to being 'on the same wavelength'" (p. 116). No wonder "patients give fuller medical histories to attuned listeners" (Halpern, 2001, p. 326). It can be easier for clients to consider and accept what you offer when what you say and how you say it feels familiar—when it better matches how they think, feel, and talk. When they feel more in sync with you, it frees them from scrutinizing every word out of your mouth with the alert suspiciousness of a border patrol agent or a teenage girl.

For the 30 years my mother-in-law, D'Aun, graced my life, I could always tell when my wife, Shelley, was talking with her on the phone. Unlike her daughter, D'Aun had a distinctive West Texas accent. Although Shelley grew up there, too, her accent is smoothed out, hardly noticeable. But her voice invariably altered a little when in conversation with D'Aun. Her cadence would shift, adapting to and subtly mirroring her mother's intonation and pacing. The transition never occurred purposefully; Shelley had no idea it was happening until I casually pointed it out one day, years into our marriage. And I'm certain that D'Aun didn't make conscious note of it, either. But with their voices paralinguistically in sync, the differences between mother and daughter were more indifferentiated than they otherwise would be. To the degree that Shelley's vocal dexterity and skill of attunement come into play in her work as a therapist, they have the potential to enhance her ability to connect with her clients and strengthen the therapeutic alliance (Imel et al., 2014; Koole & Tschacher, 2016; Palubeckas, 1981; Raingruber, 2001; Seikkula et al., 2018). And the same is true for you.

Attunement is also furthered by syncing your empathic comments with the pitch and intensity of your clients' experience. If part way through a session a client says something like "I'm at the end of my rope," you will reassure them that you're up to the challenge of being fully present for their suffering, regardless of how hopelessly desperate they feel, if you initially respond with something similar to any one of the following comments or questions. Each takes seriously and acknowledges the implications of the client's metaphor:

- "Completely spent from exhausting all your options?"
- "When everything you've tried has gone south, going on sure feels impossible."
- "Sometimes when people don't see a way forward and see everything stacked against them, thoughts of suicide start showing up. Have you noticed that happening with you?" (see Flemons & Gralnik, 2013)

However, a few of my supervisees over the years demonstrated a reluctance to fully acknowledge the depth and jagged contours of feeling that the client was describing and expressing, particularly when the question of suicidality was hovering in the room. Perhaps afraid that meeting the client on the edge would risk pushing them over it (Pollak & Ashton-James, 2018, p. 2046), they tended to temper the intensity of the client's characterization of desperation, tilting their response toward the tepid and banal. I don't remember exactly what the student therapists said, though watching and listening to the sessions from behind a one-way mirror, I wrote them down verbatim at the time. These are my best-guess reconstructions:

- "Seems you're kinda wiped out."
- "It sounds like it's been a pretty tough time for you."
- "I get that for you, the available options at the moment look fairly limited."

And some supervisees were even more out of step, attempting to fast track a shift toward hope by offering a mini pep talk or some not-so-subtle encouragement:

- "It's hard sometimes to recognize that you have more gas in the tank than you think you do. Marathon runners learn to ignore their exhaustion."
- "It sounds like you've arrived at that darkest point just before the dawn—it makes it hard to see the possibilities that are there but obscured."

Such client–therapist mismatches preclude meaningful connection and can give the client reason to get up and leave or retreat further into the loneliness of not being understood.

The third benefit that inheres in the juxtaposition of two closely related descriptions—that is, the details of the client's story and the empathic comments that you sprinkle throughout its telling—relates to the fact that the juxtaposition of the two creates what Bateson (1979/2002) referred to as a *double description*. Bateson (1979/2002) was interested in phenomena such as binocular vision, in which "two descriptions are better than one" (p. 63). In such cases, a "bonus or increment of knowing follows from *combining* information from two or more sources" (Bateson, 1979/2002, p. 63), creating information "of a sort different from what was in either source separately" (p. 19). For example, with vision, an "extra dimension to seeing"—depth perception—is introduced:

> Humans can perceive a single object in front of us with both of our eyes due to our overlapping fields of view. We cannot, however, perceive distance ahead of us with only one eye since the image on the retina of each eye is only two dimensional, on the left-right, up-down axes. It is only when the images of the two eyes are combined that the brain creates the additional sensation of depth in the forward direction. The information from our two retinas is fused to form a single image in our experience, but it is the differences in the original two images, as acknowledged and interpreted by our brains, that

generate depth perception. [Such] acts of comparison involve taking account of both the similarities and the differences between the compared objects. (Hui et al., 2008)

Bateson (1979/2002) concluded that "in principle, extra 'depth' in some metaphoric sense is to be expected whenever the information from the two descriptions is differently collected or differently coded" (p. 66).

I've heard several therapists over the years offhandedly describe a client's need "to get something off their chest" or "to vent." Characterizing clients telling their stories as a simple off-loading of information might be a fair characterization if they were speaking into the void, absent an engaged listener. Similarly, if you were to record your offering of empathic comments and hunches and then listen to them on their own, without the client's story as an orienting referent, they would sound rather wan. However, when you combine the two sources of information—the client's telling and your empathic translation—you and the client together create a context and the conditions for improved resolution and a depth of understanding to develop. As Rogers put it, "The feelings and personal meanings seem sharper when seen through the eyes of another, when they are reflected" (as cited in Kirschenbaum & Henderson, 1989b, p. 128).

I once saw a client, Georgia, who would invariably arrive at our sessions feeling, as she put it, "jumbled up"—overwhelmed and confused, with stories, reactions, impressions, and feelings swirling around her heart and mind. I didn't sit back and listen quietly, and she didn't unilaterally spew her distress; instead, we engaged in an empathy-infused back-and-forth dialogue. And from this collaborative, combined telling, we would, together, make sense of what she was going through and how she was dealing with it. As Langer (2023) underscored, "Behavior makes sense from the actor's perspective or else she or he wouldn't have done it" (p. 67).

A client of Carl Rogers (1989a), who would come to therapy feeling as disarrayed as Georgia did, offered an account of Rogers's contributions to his well-being. "Every now and again," he wrote to Rogers,

> with me in a tangle of thought and feeling, screwed up in a web of mutually divergent lines of movement, with impulses from different parts of me, and me feeling the feeling of its being all too much and suchlike—then whomp, just like a sunbeam thrusting its way through cloudbanks and tangles of foliage to spread a circle of light on a tangle of forest paths, came some comment from you. [It was] clarity, even disentanglement, an additional twist to the picture, a putting in place. Then the consequence—the sense of moving on, the relaxation. These were sunbeams. (p. 226)

The client depicted Rogers's contribution as shining down from above, piercing through his, the client's, internal confusion. Fair enough. But let's place next to this sketch a characterization informed by an understanding of double description:[1] The clarity of Rogers's confusion-slaying comment (no doubt preceded by several other empathic offerings) and the client's illumination each emerged from the comparison of their overlapping but somewhat different descriptions of the client's experience.

The two-soup redundancy—or tautology (Sundararajan, 1995)—inherent in empathic dialogue makes possible the collaborative creation of what might best be termed *empathic depth conception*—a jointly derived grasp of the client's world, a three-dimensional rendering constituted by the double description of the client's story (cf. Bohart & Greenberg, 1997b, pp. 422–423). Gendlin (1992) offered an account of how depth of meaning arises from the therapist

> listening and saying back the crux of what [the client] . . . intended to communicate. If you did just only this, . . . if you impose nothing, then what people open before you is . . . an intricate mesh of their livings and meanings. These are not on the surface. They lie always a few steps further in from the more tritely formed feelings and meanings that the person has mostly thought and felt. When this intricacy and these deeper meanings open, they are new and fresh not only [to] the therapist, but also to the person. (p. 451)

Recalling a particularly fraught time when she had felt scared, vulnerable, and disoriented, Jamison (2014) described needing people "to deliver my feelings back to me in a form that was legible. Which is a superlative kind of empathy to seek, or to supply: an empathy that rearticulates more clearly what it's shown" (p. 15).

This chapter is devoted to detailing and illustrating the skills involved in facilitating such meaningful conversations and illuminations, but first, let's talk about a few of the challenges you face in attempting to learn and/or teach these skills.

CHALLENGES TO LEARNING HOW TO EMPATHICALLY ENGAGE

In the early 1940s, when Rogers was first developing his understanding of empathy at Ohio State University, he and his students started analyzing audio recordings of their sessions, pinpointing the effects on clients of different therapist responses. Looking back at those days, Rogers (1980) noted how focused they got on "the techniques that the counselor or therapist was using. We became expert in analyzing, in very minute detail, the ebb and flow of the process in each interview, and we gained a great deal from that microscopic study" (p. 138). During this time, the teaching and research he conducted

---

[1]Yes, you're exactly right—the comparison of the client's and my accounts, juxtaposing single and double description, creates a meta double description.

and sponsored (e.g., Rogers, 1942) "centered almost exclusively on counselor techniques" (Kirschenbaum, 1979, p. 136).

Following in Rogers's footsteps, many teachers and researchers conceptualized, operationalized, and taught empathy as an interpersonal skill (e.g., Truax & Carkhuff, 1967), comprising various "microcounseling" techniques (Ivey, 1971), including "reflective listening." Often equated with empathy (Bozarth, 1997, p. 92), reflective listening became commonly identified as the "main technique of client-centered therapy" (Shlien, 1961, p. 302).

Closely following what the client is saying while simultaneously attending to tone of voice and other nonverbal indicators of affect, a reflective listener offers paraphrases of content and reflections of feeling (e.g., Ivey, 1971, pp. 57–59). According to John Shlien, reflection "is an instrument of artistic virtuosity in the hands of a sincere, intelligent, empathic listener" (as cited in Kirschenbaum & Henderson, 1989b, p. 127). However, some therapists and educators, mistakenly considering the secret sauce of empathy to be the "verbatim repetition of the client's speech" (Arnold, 2014, p. 354), advocated staying "very close to what the client has said" (Rosengren, 2009, p. 36), adding little "beyond what has already been stated" (Rosengren, 2009, p. 36). As a result, reflection became a "wooden technique of pseudo-understanding" (Rogers, 1962, p. 420, Footnote 1), which was widely criticized (Ivey, 1971, p. 61) and mercilessly caricatured (Kirschenbaum, 1979). For example, in the early 1940s, different versions of an apocryphal story began appearing, satirizing Rogers as a mindless, hapless automaton:

> Rogers is seeing a client in his office on the 10th floor of a building. The client tells Rogers that he is really depressed, and Rogers says, "Sounds like you're really depressed." The client goes on to say that he is thinking of killing himself, and Rogers responds, "You're so depressed that you're even thinking you might take your life." This "reflection" goes on and on for quite a while until the client eventually declares, "I'm so depressed I'm thinking I might jump out of that window." Rogers again reflects back, almost verbatim, what the client just said, at which point the client goes over to the window, opens it and says, "I'm so depressed, I'm going to jump out of this window." Rogers says, "You're so depressed you might jump out of that window." Exasperated, the client stands on the ledge, and the last thing out of his mouth as he jumps is, "Ahhhhhh!" Rogers, left in the office alone, repeats, "Ahhhhhh." (Neukrug, 2017; cf. Kirschenbaum, 1979, p. 135)

Rogers, who, of course, never actually lost a client in this manner (Kirschenbaum, 1979, p. 135), became "more than a little horrified" by the way his therapeutic method was distorted (Rogers, 1962, p. 420). The misunderstandings led to such "appalling consequences" that Rogers (1980) "for a number of years . . . said almost nothing about empathic listening," exclusively focusing instead on the importance of adopting an "empathic attitude" (p. 139).

Technique alone, stripped of a commitment to compassion, mindful presence, and vibrant empathic curiosity, becomes arid and empty (cf. Raingruber, 2001). Shapiro (2012), for example, criticized medical training approaches that focus on

> specific verbal and nonverbal phrases or gestures [as] . . . stand-ins for empathy: "I understand your concern"; "Your language is expressing sadness"; "I grasp that you don't want to die." Similarly, touching a shoulder or knee also reductively becomes synonymous with empathy. (p. 278)

However, attitude alone, uncoupled from the means to put it into practice, can leave you flailing, stranded with good intentions and the unrealizable desire to make a difference. To learn and implement the art of empathic engagement, you need head, heart, *and* hand. Inspiration for how to do so can be found in the world of jazz.

If you're an aspiring jazz musician, getting scales and melodic and harmonic shapes in your hands will help contain and structure your playing and improvised dialogue with other musicians (J. Decristofaro, personal communication, July 5, 2023; Sudnow, 1978). The logic and movement of such patterns, embedded in muscle memory, provide scaffolding for moment-by-moment choices of what to play. If you're an aspiring therapist, getting the techniques of empathic engagement—everything I'm covering in this chapter—in hand will help contain and shape your moment-by-moment dialogue with clients. Such patterns, embedded as background habits of framing and communication, provide scaffolding for moment-by-moment choices of what to say.

Nevertheless, for both musicians and therapists, the conscious focus on technique, which is essential for *acquiring* skills, becomes an impediment when *implementing* them. Rollo May made a similar point when comparing therapists and painters: "The therapist's situation is like that of an artist who has spent many years of disciplined study learning technique; but he knows that if specific thoughts of technique preoccupy him when he actually is in the process of painting, he has at the moment lost his vision" (as cited in Truax & Carkhuff, 1967, p. 330). Thus, it is essential to distinguish preparation from performance. As jazz educator and musician Jason Decristofaro explained,

> You get to where you understand the theory well enough and your hands know the patterned pathways thoroughly enough that when you get on stage, you don't have to think about it; you let it sit in the background like the warp, the vertical threads, of a loom. You entirely focus your attention on closely listening to, following, and playing with what the other musicians are playing and where the tune is heading. Your improvising (what I think of as the shuttling of the horizontal woof of that loom) emerges from that conversation between you and the tune and between you and the other players. (personal communication, October 15, 2024)

You can think of the ideas and practices in this chapter—and, more broadly, in the book as a whole—as a series of vertical threads, setting up the warp of the loom of empathic engagement. Once you've thought them through and practiced them enough to have them organized and embodied, you can leave them arrayed in the background as you bring your foreground focus to weaving spontaneous, improvisational conversations with your clients (cf. Nachmanovitch, 2019).

There is research evidence that empathy training improves empathy skills (Mirzaei Maghsud et al., 2020; Rautalinko et al., 2007), and there are many excellent training guides available for facilitating such learning (e.g., Clark, 2007; Egan & Reese, 2019; R. N. Goldman et al., 2021; Ivey et al., 2010). Here, I offer a streamlined way of approaching the challenge of getting up to speed, one designed to help you protect the spontaneity and humanity at the heart of empathy while avoiding the allure of defaulting to standardized riffs (e.g., Ivey et al., 2010, p. 184) or getting overwhelmed and knotted up by too many fine-grained distinctions between and within technique subcategories (see Ivey, 1971, p. 60; Rautalinko & Lisper, 2004). As you attend to the story the client is telling, you project your imagination inside of it, conjuring a first-person position from which to witness the unfolding narrative. You empathically engage by marking and verbally noting pertinent details regarding how they're relating to what they're facing—how they're making sense of it, how they're orienting to (feeling about) it, what choices they're making and actions they're taking in response to it, and what difference if any, their efforts to date have made.

EMPATHIC LISTENING

Listening is not a reaction, it is a connection. Listening to a conversation or a story, we don't so much respond as join in—become part of the action.
                      –Ursula K. Le Guin, *The Wave in the Mind* (2004)

As a Zen teacher, I do one-on-one study with students. . . . The general sense I have is that people want to be heard. They don't necessarily want answers, they don't want to be told anything, they want to be heard. So the question becomes for me, can I listen? Can I acknowledge what they're saying?
            –Bernie Glassman, *The Dude and the Zen Master* (Bridges & Glassman, 2012)

A man in one of my workshops told me and the other participants that over his long career as a family physician, he had developed the habit of barely listening to his patients, tuning them out after hearing what he estimated to be only 20% of what they had to say. Impatient with loquacious "storytellers" and ever conscious of his always-crowded waiting room, he felt compelled "to move things along." He also found it emotionally taxing "to listen to their complaining." The efforts I discussed in Chapter 4—eschewing mutuality, embracing ignorance, not presuming, and not judging—all contribute to your capacity to listen. But you can't sustain it for long if you're not also willing and able, as I mentioned in Chapter 1 and elaborated in Chapter 2, to show up and be available for your clients or patients, tolerating any discomfort or pain that may arise in you as you bear witness to their distress.

My workshop participant had found that he could both regulate his exposure to his patients' emotions and make efficient use of his limited time by beginning to formulate his response to their questions and concerns soon after they'd begun voicing their concerns. He didn't want to appear rude, so he'd stay quiet and feign attentiveness, but as soon as politely possible, he would explain his diagnosis, make recommendations, and write a script or make a referral. However, he had recently come to realize that this way of managing his appointments hadn't done him any favors. He didn't know how to sit and truly listen to anyone, he said, and he felt like his relationship with his patients had suffered.

Researchers would concur. When physicians curtail their listening, it renders them "oblivious to patients' emotional distress" (R. Epstein, 2017, p. 19). This is a common occurrence. "In one study of thoracic surgeons seeing patients with lung cancer, over 90 percent of the emotional content of conversations went unacknowledged" (R. Epstein, 2017, p. 19). The physician in my workshop was also hobbling his ability to gather pertinent information. According to Halpern (2012), patients offer "fuller medical histories to attuned listeners" (p. 235). When a listener is distracted, the lack of close attention to the speaker's meaning negatively affects the coherence of the story being told (Bavelas et al., 2000, p. 950). So how do patients and clients know that clinicians are attuned, that they are listening?

I've supervised beginning therapists who would argue that sitting forward and silently nodding while their client tells a labyrinthine story is a fine way of demonstrating engagement and showing respect. They weren't wrong, or at least not entirely. There are certainly occasions when "remaining judiciously silent" (Bohart & Greenberg, 1997b, p. 431) is a sign of sensitivity and caring. Silence is a way of "letting the patient know that some things cannot be spoken but can nevertheless be shared" (R. Epstein, 2017, p. 120).

However, I remember a particular student sitting across from a discursive client who uttered barely a word for the better part of the session. When I asked her in a postsession meeting about her reticence, she said that she thought it would be disrespectful for her to interrupt the client's soliloquy. Perhaps she had in mind the protocols at the United Nations. Delegates from each country are given an allotted time and the receptive silence necessary to assert their positions without interruption (United Nations, n.d.). However, such international gatherings are designed for each country to go on record with a prepared position they are officially espousing. A client in a therapy session is speaking spontaneously, and they are typically in search of something more than a quiet, passive audience. They aren't issued a handbook with a protocol dictating how they are to conduct themselves. Wound up or shut down, they typically want to tell their story, they want to be understood, and they want some part of their experience to change. For you to effectively use your 50 minutes (or 6 minutes if you are a physician) to facilitate that happening, your empathic listening will need to be active. This involves your "responding in a way that makes it clear that [you] . . . appreciate . . . both the meaning and the feeling behind" what the other is saying (Rogers & Farson, 1957/2021).

Reflective Listening

The term *reflective listening* derives from the metaphor of a mirror, which Rogers introduced in his 1942 book, *Counseling and Psychotherapy*. Rogers proposed that the therapist should serve as a "mirror by which the client can see himself" (Rogers & Wallen, as cited in Arnold, 2014, p. 358), offering responses that are, for the client, "a clear mirror image of the meanings and perceptions that make up his or her world of the moment" (Rogers, 1989b, p. 128). This commitment to "accurate reflection" sets the goal of a one-to-one correspondence between the client's feelings and the therapist's sayings. No wonder that in an effort to emulate Rogers's "precise and sustained fidelity to the client's emotional experience" (Arnold, 2014, p. 355), some therapists adopted the "linguistic formula" of parroting the client's words (Lieber, 1995, p. 634). Any such effort to achieve precision and accuracy is informed by a classical conception of emotion (see Barrett, 2017a) and interpersonal communication.

As I detailed in Chapter 2, an emotion is not some isolable "pure feeling" that resides inside a person in some prepackaged form, ready to be accessed, registered, and conveyed. An emotion is the brain's extemporaneous interpretation—categorization—of simple affect (Barrett, 2017a) within the context of remembered, current, and anticipated happenings and relationships. It is mind–body thinking in action, an orientation to whatever is being predicted and encountered. When a person puts a name to an emotion they're feeling, whether they're alone[2] or in conversation with others, they fold the defining capacity of language into the scenario, which influences how they're making sense of what they're feeling and how they're responding to what they're expecting and facing.

As a therapist empathically engaging with a client, you attend to the story they're telling and also to sensory indicators of how they're orienting to their experience. Listening to the details they relay, you project your imagination into the thick of things, training your eyes and ears on the manner of their telling and staying alert to how your body is registering and digesting what you're coming to understand. As you then give voice to what you're hearing and grasping and sensing, your imagination-infused articulation of the client's experience is not a mirror you're holding up to them, reflecting their feeling; it's much more like a prism, refracting their story. Bozarth (1997) once asserted that "reflection is not empathy" and "empathy is not reflection" (p. 92). I agree. Empathic listening is not reflective; it's *refractive*.

Refractive Listening

According to Bohart and Rosenbaum (1995),

> An empathic response . . . does not merely mirror back to the client what the client has just done or experienced, but carries it forward by "bouncing off it" in a creative fashion. . . . [In the] byplay that occurs between two jazz musicians improvising, . . . each takes off and goes further from where the other left off. . . . Neither musician simply repeats what the other has done, nor tries to intuit or copy in some sense what was going on in the other's mind. Empathy . . . is a carrying forward rather than somehow a copying or a representing the other's experience. (p. 12)

To be up to the improvisational challenge of refractive listening, you must be alive to the moment—mindfully aware not only of the client's words but also their meaning (Bavelas et al., 2000). You can't phone it in (see Langer, 2023, p. 174). As you listen to the person relaying their story, locating your imagination inside their first-person position, you give voice to details that

---

[2]Of course, language is learned and shared, so even if an isolated person silently names an emotion, a chorus of voices is singing along in unison.

stand out, details that together weave the fabric of their experience. Here's a brief example:

CLIENT: It's like my mind has it in for me or something. I try to stay positive, to think positive things, but then, like, subconsciously, the rug is pulled out, and then wham, I'm back feeling bad.

THERAPIST: You've been trying so hard to stay positive.

The therapist singles out and emphasizes the effort the client has been making.

CLIENT: I know, right? But it doesn't last.

The client's agreement endorses the resonance between the therapist's statement and the client's experience.

Numerous studies and several meta-analyses have established that perceived (Elliott et al., 2018) or expressed therapist empathy is reliably related to psychotherapy outcome (Norcross & Lambert, 2018; Wampold & Imel, 2015), accounting for approximately 9% of its variance (Elliott et al., 2011). Clients of more empathic therapists tend to progress more in therapy (Norcross & Lambert, 2018), perhaps because early experiences of empathy in a therapeutic relationship strengthen the working alliance (McClintock et al., 2018). Perceptions of empathy are significantly correlated with measures of the therapeutic alliance (Nienhuis et al., 2018; mean $r = 0.5$), and a strong alliance is predictive of psychotherapy outcome, at least in individual therapy (Flückiger et al., 2018). When you effectively demonstrate your empathic understanding, clients can relax their border-patrol efforts and more easily accept your comments as insider contributions rather than outsider intrusions. Then, when a therapeutic possibility is offered—say, a suggested shift in orientation to, and/or engagement with, a problem—the client can consider and digest it without having to vet it first.

THERAPIST: The rug gets pulled.

Incorporating the client's metaphor underscores the surprise element of the change.

CLIENT: And I'm back where I started.

THERAPIST: Flat on your back.

This "carries forward" (Bohart & Rosenbaum, 1995) the metaphor of a pulled rug, expressing the disoriented helplessness of falling.

CLIENT: Exactly.

THERAPIST: Which doesn't exactly inspire positive thinking.

The therapist wryly speculates on the imagined dispiriting effect of a sudden, unexpected return of feeling bad.

CLIENT: [*laughs*] No, no, it doesn't.

The client's agreement, along with the laugh, suggests that the therapist's speculation hit home.

THERAPIST: The collapse of your positive outlook took you by surprise?

This question unpacks the client's metaphor of the pulled rug: The therapist imagines that the sudden shift in outlook registered not as a dwindling but as a collapse.

CLIENT: It shouldn't have. It keeps happening.

THERAPIST: You get your hopes up that you can sustain it?

CLIENT: Stupidly, yeah.

The client's self-critical dismissiveness makes sense as a response to dashed hope.

THERAPIST: Stupid because it feels like you should know better?

CLIENT: By now, yeah.

THERAPIST: Or because you haven't yet learned how to respond effectively when the worry and the doubts first start showing up?

The therapist refracts the client's initial description of "feeling bad" into the more tangible, and thus eminently more changeable, "worry and doubts." And the question introduces the beginnings of a therapeutic suggestion—the idea that it might be possible for the client to learn to do something different in nurturing and maintaining a positive outlook. It piques the client's interest.

CLIENT: You think that's possible?

Let's back up. The metaphor of a mirror can give you the mistaken impression that there is a best empathic response, one that most purely reflects, without distortion, what the client is saying and feeling. But because emotions are categories—context-influenced interpretations of affective arousal—the relationship between body feeling and emotional experience is variable and fluid; there is no consistent one-to-one correspondence. Just as "the same emotion category involves different bodily responses" (Barrett, 2017a, p. 15), so too, the same affective arousal can be categorized and thus interpreted as different emotions. With no source feeling inside the client to locate and reflect, empathic engagement becomes an interactive construction of shared meaning and understanding (cf. Bavelas et al., 2000). This has important implications for the use of empathy in a clinical setting. Instead of searching for the right empathic reflection, you can work on offering empathic refractions that are therapeutically useful, that have a little therapeutic mustard or English on them (see Chapter 3). Empathy has a role not only in promoting change (J. C. Watson et al., 2014) but also in inviting it (Lazareva, 2020). Your professional understanding of how minds, bodies, and emotions work and your knowledge of how to invite and nurture therapeutic change can and should help determine what you highlight and refract from your client's story. Much of the therapeutic potential of empathy lives inside the gap between affect and emotion—that is, between sensation and meaning, between experience and description.

This means that when you are giving voice to your imagination's forays into and through the client's world, you have the freedom and latitude to choose emotion descriptors that the client endorses as fitting and that imply client resourcefulness and/or indirectly suggest possibilities for therapeutic change. This is "an invitation to empathise with the 'solution' part of the client/system" (Perry, 1993, p. 71). In the earlier dialogue, that's what the therapist's final question accomplishes: The phrase "haven't yet learned" implies that the return to feeling bad isn't the result of an unfortunate character trait but simply the current absence of a skill that can be acquired.

Here's another example from a session with a husband whose wife had described him over the phone to the therapist when setting up the appointment as thin-skinned, angry, and passive-aggressive:

CLIENT: My wife said that she didn't tell me what happened with the car because she "just knew" how I'd react. I was so furious she said that, I refused to talk to her for 3 days.

From the client's perspective, he had taken a principled stand and felt the need to send a message.

THERAPIST: Her prediction that you would react badly really pissed you off.

Stating the obvious was less than ideal—the client responded with a bit of attitude.

CLIENT: You think?

THERAPIST: Which you wanted her to understand.

CLIENT: Without question.

THERAPIST: It hurts when someone you care about worries about your ability to handle upsetting news.

The therapist refracted the client's *fury* as *hurt* and the wife's accusatory prediction as an expression of worry. The client accepted both:

CLIENT: Of course.

THERAPIST: Her opinion of you obviously means so much.

Now, the intensity of the man's fury was a measure of the intensity of his caring for his wife.

CLIENT: Yeah, I guess it does.

THERAPIST: Makes sense, then, that you needed a healthy chunk of time to collect yourself.

The wife had viewed the husband's 3-day "silent treatment" as the petulant expression of a passive-aggressive man intent on punishing her; the therapist's refraction classified it as a healthy commitment to regaining balance. The man agreed:

CLIENT: I did.

The therapist's refractions helped establish a direction for their work together. The client became interested in learning how to continue caring about what his wife thought of him and to develop skills for managing this sensitivity differently. In addition, he recognized the wisdom of drawing back from conflictual situations so he could regroup, and he was interested in learning how he might shorten the time it took to do so.

Langer (2023) pointed out that "every negative ascription has an equally potent but oppositely valanced alternative," which means it can also be framed positively: "Someone who is gullible is also trusting; someone who is grim is also serious" (p. 106); someone who is anxious is sensitive and alert; someone who is afraid is prioritizing safety; someone who is angry is temporarily marking a clear boundary between self and someone or something threatening or irritating; someone who is disappointed or disheartened has a clear conception of how things should be; someone who is stuck is, for the moment, poised in stillness. Because an emotion category is an indicator of how the person is orienting to their circumstances, relabeling or reframing—revalancing—it can shift the parameters within which goals are set and solutions are sought and found (cf. Watzlawick et al., 1974). It is easier for a man to change if he is hurt rather than furious; if he is sensitive to, rather than angrily dismissive of, his wife's opinion; if he is committed to taking the necessary time to collect himself rather than caught up in passive-aggressive punishment.

Let's circle back and take another look at the client whose positivity crashed and burned. Recall what he said:

CLIENT: It's like my mind has it in for me or something. I try to stay positive, to think positive things, but then, like, subconsciously, the rug is pulled out, and then wham, I'm back feeling bad.

And recall what the therapist said about the client's significant and sustained efforts:

THERAPIST: You've been trying so hard to stay positive.

This comment nicely teed up the possibility of asking a therapeutically valanced follow-up question:

THERAPIST: Do you typically go all in when you set out to accomplish something important?

However, other empathic responses to the client's initial statement were possible, each with a little therapeutic spin on them:

THERAPIST: It's like your subconscious has a different agenda, one you don't yet understand.

There's that *yet* doing its magic again. A not-yet-understood agenda could give rise to current misunderstandings (e.g., "My mind is malevolent") but also future discoveries (e.g., "There's something to be learned about how things went south").

THERAPIST: It hurts when hope takes a big hit like that.

The client didn't mention hope; the therapist infers that the client's efforts to think positively had been fueled by it. Hope that's taken a hit may be shaken to its core, but it's still there to be accessed. Another possibility:

THERAPIST: Thinking positively was making a difference, but you painfully discovered that something more is needed to sustain the change.

Before the rug was pulled, the client was onto something, and change was underway. The next step would be to regroup and discover and implement the "something more."

I talked earlier about the importance of attuning to and matching the intensity of what the client is communicating as you bear witness to their suffering. When you therapeutically refract what the client is telling you, you strive to stay in sync with their experience while inferring their implicit strengths and resources. You introduce possibilities for change via implication, not imposition. If you move too fast, getting ahead of where the client is, you can most often count on them correcting you. That's the beauty of empathic *engagement*—you're able to continually adjust your understanding and what you say next in response to the client's responses to what you just said.

ERROR CORRECTION

Life is about . . . managing expectations, repeat business, and error correction.
—Steven Soderbergh, in *Talk Easy* (Fragoso, 2024)

Failures provide a certain kind of feedback that is then used in . . . error correction. With this simple loop in place, knowing that something doesn't work can be as valuable as knowing that it does.
—Stuart Firestein, *Failure* (2016)

I had little hesitancy in doing a good deal of empathic guessing, for I had learned that though [the client] . . . might not respond in any discernible way when I was right in my inferences, he would usually let me know by a negative shake of his head if I was wrong.
—Betty D. Meador & Carl R. Rogers, *Person-Centered Therapy* (1984, p. 166)

Approaching your clients with humility, not presuming that you know their experience, you recognize and accept that every empathic refraction you offer is a guess and thus an experiment. This means that you need to always be checking in with the client to get a read on how your empathic understanding is developing (Bozarth, 2009, p. 109). "*Clients are better judges of the degree of empathy than are therapists. . . .* Perhaps, if we wish to become better therapists, we should let our clients tell us whether we are understanding them accurately" (Rogers, 1975, p. 6; see also Fraser & Solovey, 2007, p. 70). How does this work? Gendlin (1992) offered an account:

> A person says something; one responds by saying back its crux. The person hears it said back. It isn't quite what the person intended. The person corrects it. The therapist accepts the correction (of course, since it is the client's meaning that is to be grasped here). The client hears it. Yes, now, that is mostly right, but there is still a little wrinkle that wasn't heard. That too is said, heard, and said back. Then the client says the next thing, and again it is said back and the saying-back is corrected, until the client feels heard. (p. 451)

You offer an empathic refraction, and the client provides the feedback necessary to help you determine whether you're on track. It is the two of you together, collaborating, that creates the depth of empathic understanding I spoke about earlier. Nevertheless, as a process, empathy is always

> inevitably incomplete. . . . The session is directed principally not by therapist interventions but by the feed-back from the [client]. . . . The therapist cannot understand fully or express exactly. But if her/his attempts . . . are close enough, they will evoke a response which will help therapist and clients proceed further. (Perry, 1993, p. 72)

When what you offer fits for the client, it helps them recognize the quality of your listening and the fact that you're empathically grasping something of their experience. Their verbal and/or nonverbal acknowledgment of this fit helps you, in turn, recognize that you're on track. Whenever they imply or say something like "Yes," "Right," "Exactly," or "Nicely put," you know you've taken another step into the interior of their world:

CLIENT: My husband and kids are ready for me to get the operation yesterday. But I'm 79. I've had a good life. And I'm so very, very tired.

THERAPIST: Your family isn't ready to say goodbye.

CLIENT: They aren't ready, no.

THERAPIST: But it sounds like you are.

This wasn't quite correct.

CLIENT: I don't know that I'm ready to say goodbye, but I am ready to stop fighting.

When the client lets you know that your offering doesn't fit, they give you the opportunity to question and correct your assumptions before trying again with a more nuanced refraction:

THERAPIST: Too tired to keep fighting the cancer, but I imagine also too tired to fight with your family about the surgery.

Sometimes, you get an empathic sense of something the client has not explicitly said or perhaps even formulated, something "at the periphery of [their] awareness" (Elliott et al., 2011, p. 48). The therapist's final comment brought into foreground focus for the client a conundrum she'd been worrying about but hadn't been able to clearly articulate, not to herself and certainly not to her husband or kids. Could she muster the strength necessary, she wondered, to stand up to her family and convince them she didn't have the strength necessary to pursue more treatment?

Your embrace of trial-and-error learning, a signature feature of empathic engagement (Halpern, 2001, p. 73), is essential for improving the perceived accuracy, and thus the granularity, of your imaginings. It also reassures the client of your commitment to them and to the empathic process (MacFarlane, 2013, p. 48).

> The therapist is at times bound to misunderstand or not grasp the client's experience. When the therapist . . . tries to grasp empathically how he or she has failed to grasp the client's world, the client realizes the therapist is with him or her. (Greenberg & Elliott, 1997, p. 175)

As Halpern (2012) put it, "Inviting the patient to let you know what you are missing or getting wrong is a very important way to build trust and a therapeutic alliance" (p. 237).

I once saw a client, Jacqueline, who let me know—in no uncertain terms—what I was getting wrong. However, despite welcoming her feedback and making adjustments to what I was offering in response to what she said, I failed to come across to her as credible or helpful. As Elliott et al. (2011) noted, certain clients "may find the usual expressions of empathy too intrusive, . . . too directive . . . [or] too foreign," which means you "need to know when—and when not—to respond empathically" (p. 48). It is important to use your "perspective-taking skills" to help you "respect [your] . . . client's boundaries" and "provide an optimal therapeutic distance" (Elliott et al., 2011, p. 48). Or, in the words of my good friend Kate, offering advice to her 16-year-old when he was being an oblivious teenage boy, "Read the room!"

I wish the day I saw Jacqueline I'd had Elliott et al.'s (2011) counsel in mind and Kate's voice in my ear. Jacqueline hadn't spoken to her son since his wedding a year earlier when she'd accused his new wife of turning him against her. Agonized by a cold silence that she blamed on the young couple but particularly the wife, she'd come to me hoping to lay the foundations for a rapprochement. I moved too fast and presumed too much.

DOUGLAS: Given the pain you've endured, I imagine that even contemplating the building of a connecting bridge [to your son and daughter-in-law] feels like a considerable emotional risk.

JACQUELINE: [*derisively*] Emotional risk?! You have to be kidding. . . . There is *no* risk whatsoever! Pain? Oh, yes. There's nothing more painful than losing a child.

I could feel the immediacy of and sense the protection offered by Jacqueline's righteous fury, but I didn't recognize until later, until she'd already dismissed me as clueless, that during our session, she had consistently rejected, outright, any refraction I offered that suggested or implied that she felt any sort of vulnerability. Fuming and blaming felt safe; exposure definitively did not.

Rogers (1962) recognized the importance of staying on top of the way the client is responding to what you're offering. "I have learned," he said, that "empathy can be perceived as lack of involvement; that an unconditional regard on my part can be perceived as indifference; that warmth can be perceived as a threatening closeness, that real feelings of mine can be perceived as false" (Rogers, 1962, p. 422). In keeping with this sensitivity, Bohart and Greenberg (1997b) explored the question of whether empathy can prove harmful, citing one study that concluded, "Therapists who are actively empathic, supportive, and involved are actually counter-effective with clients who are reactant against authority, poorly motivated, suspicious, and highly sensitive" (p. 431; see also Elliott et al., 2018; Norcross & Lambert, 2018, p. 312).

I would make the point more broadly, sans pointing finger. If you're working with someone who, for whatever reason, finds it threatening to be in conversation with you, then your empathic efforts to understand and your therapeutic efforts to help can easily go awry. The first order of business is protecting their boundaries (Elliott et al., 2011, p. 48) and ensuring their safety (cf. Linehan, 2020), which will probably involve taking a step back from articulating the sense you're making of their experience. At such times, "it may be more empathic," as Bohart and Greenberg (1997b) suggested, "to keep a respectful distance" (p. 432), even "remaining judiciously silent for a time" (p. 431).

Had I been quicker on my feet with Jacqueline, I perhaps could have, midsession, pivoted away from imagining her emotional risk and toward offering an appreciation of the strength and courage involved in reaching out to her son through the incredible pain she'd endured. This might have allowed us to discuss ways of approaching him and his wife that were more and less likely to succeed. But I was too slow on the uptake, so we never got there; Jacqueline decided not to schedule another session.

ASKING QUESTIONS AND FLOATING HUNCHES

Empathy comes from asking the right questions.
—Ron Perry, *Empathy–Still at the Heart of Therapy* (1993, p. 69)

Empathy isn't just listening, it's asking the questions whose answers need to be listened to. Empathy requires inquiry as much as imagination.
—Leslie Jamison, *The Empathy Exams* (2014)

Empathy can reach to areas of the person that he [or she] is not fully aware of.

–Alfred Margulies, *The Empathic Imagination* (1989)

You may remember from Chapter 1 that I'm from Canada? And perhaps you're aware that we Canadians are noted (okay, mocked) for our rising inflection at the end of declarative sentences? So that even when we're saying something definitive, we sound like we're asking a question? Such a stereotype, eh? (I would apologize for perpetuating the stereotype, but saying "sorry" would only reinforce yet another one.)

Everything having to do with empathy works best if it has a little Eau de Canada spritzed onto it, even if you're not from there and even if, when you speak, your end-of-sentence intonation doesn't rise. I said earlier that all your offerings in empathic conversations are guesses, experiments. Suffused with a nonpresuming humility, with a healthy respect for what you don't—and can't—know about the other (Elliott et al., 2018), empathy is less about knowing than it is about wondering. It is characterized by a "questioning desire" to understand (Rogers, as cited in Kirschenbaum & Henderson, 1989b, p. 128), to make sense of the other's skills, habits, affect, beliefs, regrets, choices, reasons, efforts, worries, constraints, motivations, proclivities, and so on. Satisfying that desire involves probing areas of the client's experience that aren't immediately present in the initial telling of their story.

Watch just about any movie or television show depicting a therapy session, and you'll likely hear the clinician at some point ask the client, "How does that make you feel?" As much as I cringe every time I hear this question mindlessly intoned, and even though I have never asked it myself, perhaps there's a reason it dominates the public's (and screenwriters') perception of what therapists want to know. The question itself isn't inherently bad, just woefully incomplete. Halpern (2012) put it this way:

> Many research studies and medical educators presume that the cognitive aim of clinical empathy is to help the physician label the patient's emotion type correctly—recognizing for example, when a patient is angry or worried. However, I would argue that this labeling is only a very beginning step. It is often fairly obvious that a patient is angry or sad, but what needs to be understood is what, in particular, his anger or sadness *is about*. (p. 232, italic in original)

Hearing how a client feels about some circumstance helps you learn a little about how they're orienting to it. But to get a three-dimensional, first-person sense of how they experience themselves fitting into the story they're telling, you need a more elaborated grasp of the intra- and interpersonal contextual details informing their affective response (cf. Elliott et al., 2018). That's where questions come into play, informed by your empathic curiosities:

- How has the client been making sense of the circumstance, predicament, or conundrum in which they find themself?
- What have been the physical and emotional effects of their involvement in the situation?
- What have the person and others chosen to do in response to the situation, and what has been the result of their efforts?
- Who and what has been helpful?
- Who and what has been unhelpful?
- In what ways have the choices of the client and others been limited?
- In what ways have or could the client's and others' choices been expanded?
- What is the context for what's happening now? How does the current scenario fit into a more encompassing story, one that began before the immediate present and/or involves more than the immediate players?
- Projecting into the future, what are the client's and others' predictions? What expectancies are informing their current experience?
- What does the client not yet understand?
- What does the client want or feel the need to learn?

As your empathic understanding gets fleshed out by the client's answers to such questions, the fine-grained, affect-rich details of their world come into enhanced focus. The more details you get in hand and are able to confirm with the client, the more they can trust you as an insider. And by connecting dots—each of the various points of confirmation—you establish a constellation of understanding beyond which to project your embodied imagination, offering hunches that venture into areas of the person's experience that they haven't yet articulated and may not have previously considered.

Your out-loud conjecturing isn't a detached working out of what the client's experience is likely to be; it makes possible the interpersonal error correction necessary for you to get a feel for the relational logic of how the client is relating to themself and their circumstances. Neither are you imagining, "I'm guessing that this is what I would be feeling or doing if *I* were in this situation." As I explained in Chapter 2, in-the-shoes empathizing tethers your imagination to *your* history and sensibility, leaving the client's relatively untouched and unappreciated.

By projecting your metaphoric imagination into the heart of *being* the client, you get a vicarious felt sense (Gendlin, 1981) of their circumstances, with their history and their relationships with significant others. Extrapolating from the details you've established with the client's feedback, you float hunches about what you imagine could be the case, what the client might have been (or currently might be) feeling, avoiding, attempting, choosing, deciding, and so on. When you give voice to such conjectures, offering them up to the client for feedback, you invite the two of you to consider refractive possibilities—the wellspring of therapeutic change.

A man, Ted, in a strained marriage, scheduled an appointment at his wife's insistence. She was concerned, he said, about his impatience with her and the kids, which she attributed to his feeling overwhelmed, anxious, and unhappy. Early in the session, Ted began itemizing some of his irritations with his wife.

TED: My wife overreacts to certain things—like she'll hyperfocus on someone's tone.

I was more interested in his reaction to such overreactions, so I floated a hunch:

DOUGLAS: Which would be uncomfortable if that someone were to be you.

Ted paused to agree before completing the point he was making.

TED: [*laughs*] True, but also when I see her in a social situation . . .

DOUGLAS: Zeroing in.

TED: Yes, [focusing] on whether or not somebody may, you know, hold eye contact with her, if somebody said hi to her . . .

DOUGLAS: Was somehow disrespectful.

TED: Exactly.

Orienting refractively, I put a little therapeutic mustard on some of my questions and hunches:

DOUGLAS: Your wife is sensitive to being slighted. Is she sensitive in other ways, too?

My question served as a segue from problem to possibility (cf. O'Hanlon & Bertolino, 1998): Sensitivity can manifest as prickliness, but it is also a key ingredient of responsiveness and engaged presence.

TED: She's very observant of the world around us.

DOUGLAS: You mentioned earlier that *you're* sensitive. I imagine that's a place where you guys have been able to connect.

A hunch involves more of a commitment than a question because you risk being wrong. I could have asked, "Does the fact that you're both sensitive contribute at all to a connection with your wife?" If he said no, his denial wouldn't have reflected negatively on my degree of understanding of his experience. But by floating it as a hunch, I was not just sketching an idea; I was offering a prediction. His response was then not only a comment on whether the idea was right but also an evaluation of whether *I* was right. As it happened, I was.

TED: We do connect on a lot of stuff. . . . I think we're both very sensitive, yes, and I think early on, I think that was probably one of the reasons that we really understood each other very well. [But then] a lot of our conflict arises from me not seeing the importance of something that she sees as very, very important.

DOUGLAS: Not seeing or not acknowledging?

If Ted simply didn't see the importance of something that mattered so much to his wife, it would imply that he was checked out or oblivious; however, if he disagreed about why it should be important and so was reluctant to acknowledge it, it opened an avenue for change. He could, for example, become empathically curious about why she cared so much, allowing him to find and acknowledge some legitimacy in her perspective.

TED: It's just that, you know, she's reacting very strongly. I hate seeing her upset.

DOUGLAS: So . . . she sensitively responds to something that she takes issue with, and you—what?—you attempt to downplay it in order to keep her from being so upset and to keep you from getting stressed?

TED: Yeah, but it never works.

DOUGLAS: You're just trying to calm everything, everybody, down.

TED: Which she objects to.

My refraction classified his efforts, however ineffectual they were, as well-meaning. This, too, had some mustard on it—it leaves room for finding a more helpful way of putting his positive intent into practice.

Sometimes, it helps to project your imagination into the position of another character in the story and float a hunch that you predict would resonate with them:

DOUGLAS: I would imagine that your wife feels like what you're doing is downplaying her legitimacy, and she takes issue with your tone or with your efforts or something.

TED: [*laughs*] You must know my wife.

I didn't—only in my imagination.

DOUGLAS: Which is all the more upsetting given your intent.

In the final section of this chapter—Both–And Empathizing—I return to the skill of shifting back and forth between different embodied perspectives. First, though, let's talk about ensuring the interactivity of your engagement with clients by developing your capacity to get a word in edgewise.

INTERLACING

[Being empathic] means frequently checking with [the client] . . . as to the accuracy of your sensings, and being guided by the responses you receive.
—Carl R. Rogers, *Empathic* (1975, p. 4)

Say back bit *by* bit *what the person tells you. Don't let the person say more than you can take in and say back. Interrupt, say back, and let the person go on.*
—Eugene T. Gendlin, *Focusing* (1981, p. 120)

I told you earlier about the student who considered interrupting her talkative client to be disrespectful. I told her that given the Latin roots of the word *interrupt* (from *inter*, "between," and *rumpere*, "to break," meaning "to break into"), I had to agree with her. I, too, want to avoid "breaking into" clients' stories. My goal is for clients to experience my engagement with them as an interlacing (from *inter*, "between," and *lacier*, "to tie," meaning "to unite by crossing laces"), as an interweaving of my voice with theirs—a Bach-like two-part invention. The more often you offer refractions, the more guiding feedback you'll get from the client, which, in turn, will improve the resolution of your developing understanding and your connection with the client:

> The more frequently the therapist responds to the client, even if only with an "um-hmm," the greater the likelihood that a high level of accurate empathy will be perceived and communicated. . . . [Such] responsiveness seems to ensure that any errors in empathy by the therapist will be corrected immediately. . . . Research also indicates that the specificity or concreteness of the therapist's response is related to both the level of accurate empathy and the level of patient engagement. (Truax & Carkhuff, 1967, p. 287)

But balance is important. If your client is less than thrilled by how active you are in your active listening, you'll need to listen to that and adapt accordingly.

You can get a feel for the pace of empathic interlacing by practicing outside of the therapy room. The next time some story-spinning person you've never met corners you at a party, instead of bewailing your fate and looking for someone to rescue you, seize the opportunity to experiment. Interlace and learn.

Alternatively, and less interactively, you might go to YouTube and find a monologue from a show you've been watching, say the character Carmy—Carmen Berzatto—on *The Bear* (Storer et al., 2022), opening his soul at an Al-Anon meeting (FX Networks, 2022). Play the clip through a couple of times to get a feel for the whole of it, projecting your imagination inside the world of the show and the embodied presence of the character at that point in the story. Then start again from the top and, pausing the video at different intervals—sometimes more, sometimes less, often—give voice to what seems to be the gist or crux (Gendlin, 1992, p. 451) of what the person is facing and how they're orienting to it.

Of course, the result would make for horrible television, and it doesn't begin to resemble an actual conversation; however, the exercise can give you a taste for empathically shifting into the character's world, comment by comment, step by step. In his monologue in Season 1, Episode 8 of *The Bear* (Storer et al., 2022), Carmen talks about his relationship with his dead brother, Michael. My inserted empathic refractions are in square brackets:

> My name's Carmen. My uh, my brother's an addict, my brother was an addict. [Was an addict—it takes a while for the reality of his death to sink in.] . . . My brother could make you feel confident in yourself. [He could build you up.] You know like when I was nervous, I was scared, I wouldn't want to do something, he'd always tell me to just face it. [You just knew he had your back.] . . . He was loud, and he was hilarious, and he had this amazing ability, he could just, he could walk into a room, and he could take the temperature of it instantly [An outsize presence, yet he was also sensitive and tuned in.] . . . I'm not built like that. [Not bigger than life like that, but how about the sensitivity?] I didn't have a lot of friends growing up. [You were more of a loner.] I had a stutter when I was a kid. I was scared to speak half the time. [With a stutter, it would have been, I imagine, way too risky to draw attention to yourself.] And I got shitty grades because I couldn't pay attention in school. [Sitting in class must have been torture.] I didn't get into college. [That option was closed off.] I didn't have any girlfriends. [Also too risky?] I don't think I'm funny. [Your brother was a hard act to follow.] I always thought my brother was my best friend, like we just knew everything about each other. [To know someone and be known like that makes it possible to face the world.] Except, everybody thought he was their best friend, you know? [I guess if everybody's special, no one is.] He was that magnetic. [He drew people to him.] And, um, I didn't know my brother was using drugs. What does that say? [If you didn't know something as important as that about him, what else did he keep from you? What else didn't you know?] As we got older, I realized I didn't know anything about him, really. [He was a mystery, a cipher.] (FX Networks, 2022, 0:01–2:52)

As I said earlier, you aren't serving as a mirror, so you aren't trying to make correct reflections; you're simply looking to offer refractions that aren't wrong.[3] And because of the classificatory nature of emotions and language in general, when the client agrees with one of your empathic comments, this doesn't mean you were "accurate." There is no direct line between the words you've uttered and some insular, preformed emotion that was residing fully formed inside the client's body. Rather, the client's agreement indicates a degree of fit or resonance between their and your respective ways of classifying and articulating their experience. So each time you pause the video, formulate and articulate a refraction with the idea that if the character could hear what you're saying, they'd look over and nod. Stay alert to the possibility that they'd look over and shake their head in disagreement ("No, it wasn't too risky to have a girlfriend") or puzzlement ("Cipher? What the hell's a cipher? I didn't go to college, remember?") and adjust your idea or vocabulary, accordingly.

Obviously, YouTube practice sessions with character monologues won't provide you with the interactive experience of noting and refractively responding to the other's affirming and error-correcting feedback; for that, you'll need to head out to another party or, of course, at some point, bring what you're learning into the therapy room.

By interlacing empathic contributions throughout the client's narrative, you alter the rhythm and course of its unfolding. The back-and-forth nature of the interaction—the client's telling, your refracting, the client's endorsing or correcting what you say, your incorporating their feedback in your subsequent refraction, and so on—establishes an expectation and enacts a practice of turn-taking (see Gardner et al., 2009; Goodwin & Heritage, 1990; Sacks et al., 1974). Each of you successively takes the floor from and then cedes it to the other. Let's take a look at this in action.

I saw a client, Noreen, who told me she struggled terribly to throw anything away. Things in the house had piled up so much that her teenage son, Troy, was now too embarrassed to bring even his best friend home. I asked her for an example or two of the things she'd been holding onto.

NOREEN: Troy asked me to sew him a sash for a Halloween costume. I have the perfect piece of fabric, except it is like a third again too long and needs to be cut. But it feels like if I do that, something bad will happen.

DOUGLAS: It needs to be shorter, but cutting it feels ominous.

---

[3]Bateson (1972/2000) explained that in cybernetic (feedback) circuits, there is "a difference between 'being right' and 'not being wrong'" (p. 411).

Empathic comments invite feedback. Clients typically let you know whether they agree with what you said, and they sometimes go on to elaborate or refine what they were saying:

NOREEN: Yeah, but also, like, if I do [cut it], I'll mess it up, or maybe later I'll need the whole length of it for something else.

When there's an expectation of turn-taking, every response is also an invitation for the other to subsequently take the floor:

DOUGLAS: A pressure not to mess with it, to preserve it.

The social convention of turn-taking potentiates two key features of refractive interlacing, both of them rhetorical skills made available when you embrace your role as "a conversational artist—an architect of the dialogical process—whose expertise is [as] . . . *a participant-facilitator of the therapeutic conversation*" (H. Anderson & Goolishian, 1992, p. 27). The first feature: It is possible for you, gradually, over the course of several conversational turns, to acknowledge the client's circumstances and their response but also, if only implicitly, to make mention of the client's strengths and resources and/or the possibility of change. In so doing, you can steer the conversation in the direction of the client's therapeutic goal. I think of this skill as a form of what Buckminster ("Bucky") Fuller called *trim tabbing*:

> Giant oceangoing tankers need a giant rudder to make them turn. But engineers discovered that it takes too much energy to turn the giant rudder. Instead, they came up with the trim tab, a tiny rudder attached to the big rudder. The little rudder turns the big rudder and the big rudder turns the ship. (Bridges & Glassman, 2012, p. 45)

Successive empathic refractions can serve as a series of trim-tab adjustments—small, subtle movements that begin altering the client's experience, understanding, and expectancy regarding their sense of self, their pain, and their capacity to change.

An elegant example of this step-by-step therapeutic shuffle can be found in Milton Erickson's engagement with his 3-year-old son, Robert, after the boy fell down some stairs, cutting open his lip and knocking a tooth into his upper jaw. Erickson (as cited in Haley, 1986) described how he responded: "His mother and I went to his aid. A single glance at him lying on the ground screaming, his mouth bleeding profusely and blood spattered on the pavement, revealed that this was an emergency requiring prompt and adequate measures" (p. 189). Erickson's first communication was an attuned, empathic acknowledgment of Robert's pain. "No effort was made to pick him up. Instead, as he paused for breath for fresh screaming, I told him quickly, simply, sympathetically and emphatically, 'That hurts awful, Robert. That hurts terrible'" (p. 189).

Erickson didn't claim understanding; he showed it.

> Right then, without any doubt, my son knew that I knew what I was talking about. He could agree with me and he knew that I was agreeing completely with him. Therefore he could listen respectfully to me, because I had demonstrated that I understood the situation fully. (p. 189)

Just as Erickson didn't rush to pick Robert up and cradle him, he also didn't attempt to counter his experience and expression of pain and fear (e.g., "Shh, shh, stop crying—it's okay, you're okay"), opting instead to further establish, by way of a prediction, that he was in sync with his son's circumstances:

> Then I told Robert, "And it will keep right on hurting." In this simple statement, I named his own fear, confirmed his own judgment of the situation, demonstrated my good intelligent grasp of the entire matter and my entire agreement with him, since right then he could foresee only a lifetime of anguish and pain for himself. (Haley, 1986, p. 190)

He then offered a hunch about what Robert desperately wanted.

> The next step for him and for me was to declare, as he took another breath, "And you really wish it would stop hurting." Again, we were in full agreement and he was ratified and even encouraged in this wish. And it was *his* wish, deriving entirely from within him and constituting his own urgent need. (Haley, 1986, p. 190, italics in original)

It was only at that point, after clearly demonstrating his empathic grasp, that Erickson offered Robert the opportunity to begin shifting his expectancy.

> With the situation so defined, I could then offer a suggestion with some certainty of its acceptance. This suggestion was, "Maybe it will stop hurting in a little while, in just a minute or two." This was a suggestion in full accord with his own needs and wishes, and, because it was qualified by a "maybe it will," it was not in contradiction to his own understandings of the situation. Thus he could accept the idea and initiate his responses to it. (Haley, 1986, p. 190)

I made some analogous trim-tab adjustments in my conversation with Noreen. She told me that in addition to finding herself unable to cut the fabric for Troy's sash, she held onto just about everything, including packing materials from new purchases.

NOREEN: I got a new phone a couple of weeks ago, and it came in this really nice box. I still have it.

DOUGLAS: It's so hard to throw out something so well constructed.

My comment acknowledged Noreen's feeling and behavior, but it also refracted them, normalizing the difficulty of treating as trash something so aesthetically pleasing. She agreed but clarified that her problem wasn't so simple:

NOREEN: Yeah, the box is nice, but the old phone isn't—the screen's cracked—and I can't let *it* go, either. It's so frustrating, so ridiculous.

Noreen was dismissive of herself, of what she considered a stubborn and nonsensical incapacity. My response resonated with her exasperation and refracted the holding on as a kind of loyalty:

DOUGLAS: So irritating. Can't give up on it . . .

NOREEN: No.

And then helpless loyalty became willful, determined loyalty by swapping *can't* with *won't*:

DOUGLAS: Won't give up on it.

NOREEN: I'm like, maybe I could get it repaired and have it as a backup for Troy in case he loses his.

My framing Noreen as a loyal and determined person wasn't blatant. I wasn't congratulating her; I was acknowledging how frustrated she was by her tendency to hang on to stuff. But little by little, trim-tab refraction by trim-tab refraction, I sprinkled the implication of legitimacy, agency, and potential into the conversation. You can see the beginnings of the effect of this in Noreen's response to my comment. Her tone was still self-critical, but she was recognizing and acknowledging that there was indeed a legitimate logic underpinning her holding onto the old phone. Her behavior wasn't irrational; it was making sense (Langer, 2023, p. 67). By the end of the session, Noreen and I were agreeing that she had the potential to become a female MacGyver.[4] The thought of that gave her "so much joy" because since she was a child, she'd always identified with the ability to "kind of pull things together and make things work."

Refractive interlacing has a second feature: It provides the rhetorical means for pivoting and segueing to a different topic. Given the back-and-forth rhythm of empathic dialogues, when the client pauses to agree with one of your refractions, they affirm that the two of you are on the same page and hand the floor back to you. This makes it possible for you to use your turn to steer or venture

---

[4]The titular main character of a long-running television series (Winkler & Rich, 1985–1992). MacGyver invented hacks for fixing things and solving problems.

in any number of potentially therapeutic directions, confident that the client, feeling aligned, will likely accompany you. When the client considers you an insider, your therapeutic contributions are less likely to be scrutinized as outside intrusions.

Noreen told me that she spent much of her time in what she described as a "micro kind of world." Staying focused on details, along with drinking alcohol and taking her prescribed benzodiazepine, kept her panic somewhat in check.

NOREEN: But then when I . . . step back, and I see what I'm surrounded by, then I'm feeling crushed by all of the stuff, . . . and then that's even more crushing and makes me feel just completely overwhelmed.

DOUGLAS: You take in the big picture, it feels suffocating.

Noreen had earlier mentioned having trouble breathing when she felt panicky. She confirmed my comment.

NOREEN: Yes.

This time, I offered a hunch, with which she also agreed.

DOUGLAS: Kinda makes you wanna keep your head down.

NOREEN: [*laughs*] Totally. When I see the bigger picture, then I realize, like, what I've kind of done to myself.

With Noreen again concurring and again returning the floor to me, I used my turn to pivot to an exploration of what she had done to resourcefully address her problem, starting with her decision to make an appointment.

DOUGLAS: So what got you to the idea, "Let me, let me find a different way of solving my problem than just doing more of what I'm doing," like, how did you arrive at [the idea of] reaching out to me?

This use of empathic comments to set up conversational pivot points is particularly helpful when you have more than one client in the room, whether you're meeting with a couple, family, or group.

BOTH-AND EMPATHIZING

The test of a first-rate intelligence is the ability to hold two opposed ideas in the mind at the same time, and still retain the ability to function.

—F. Scott Fitzgerald, *The Crack-Up* (1936, para. 2)

That two people's experiences could differ so drastically, yet both be true and deep, is maybe the most important lesson I've ever learned.

–Jamil Zaki, *The War for Kindness* (2019)

Bloom (2016) pointed out that you can't sympathetically resonate (he said "empathize")

> with more than one or two people at the same time. Try it. Think about someone you know who's going through a difficult time and try to feel what she or he is feeling. Feel that person's pain. Now at the same time do this with someone else who's in a difficult situation, with different feelings and experiences. Can you simultaneously empathize [resonate] with two people? If so, good, congratulations. Now add a third person to the mix. Now try ten. (p. 33)

Empathic engagement is different from Bloom's characterization of sympathetic resonance. He's correct that if you had two or more clients in the room together, you wouldn't be able to *feel with* each and all of them simultaneously. Nor would you want to: Affective muddle is not conducive to empathic imagining or therapeutic change. You can, however, respectively develop an idiosyncratic, felt sense of each client's unique first-person experience, keeping it distinct from the other(s) and keeping yourself from getting confused, even when the stories overlap.

When working with couples and families, it isn't uncommon for two or more people to offer descriptions of the "same" event that directly contradict each other. At such times, you don't need to nail down what "really happened." As I discussed in Chapter 2, there is no perspective-free, neutral vantage (Maibom, 2022) from which to encounter and resolve conflicting accounts. Instead, as when reading Lawrence Durrell's (1957) *The Alexandria Quartet* or watching Akira Kurosawa's (1950) *Rashomon*, you adopt what Becvar and Becvar (2013) called a *both–and* perspective (p. 383). You let go of yearning for a singular, objective truth, embracing instead a multifaceted appreciation and acceptance of *both* the stories' common elements *and* their nonresolvable differences. As F. Scott Fitzgerald (1936) might have said if he had been a family or group therapist, "It takes first-rate empathic skill to be able to hold two (or more) opposed (or divergent) stories in mind at the same time and still retain the ability to join with each storyteller and nonjudgmentally refract their version of events."

Everything you know about empathically engaging with individuals is relevant and applicable to working with groupings of people—systems—whether couples, families, or groups. However, interpersonal complexities come into play when your empathic listening is public, when clients are monitoring and comparing your way of relating to each of them relative to the other(s). When you first meet alone with an individual client, they are working out, largely under the surface, whether they feel safe speaking with you, safe to be frank and self-reflective and open—vulnerable—in front of you. They are determining if they can trust that you will respect and not judge them and that you can and will be patient, present, and resourceful.

Now, if you were to invite that same person into a conjoint session with their partner or family or into a group therapy session, they would, in addition, be assessing if they can trust that you'll be fair, that you won't unduly expose their limitations or vulnerabilities to the other(s), causing them to lose face, and you won't side with someone else against them:

> For therapists used to working with individuals, there is a particular difficulty when working with families and systems. Getting involved too deeply in empathy with one person can skew understanding of the system as a whole, and endanger engagement with the group. For example, it can be a risk to appear to empathise too much with an adolescent when the parents may see this as taking sides against their point of view. (Perry, 1993, p. 65)

Young therapists are particularly susceptible to being suspiciously perceived by parents as problematically pro-kid, just as older therapists are at risk of being suspiciously perceived by teenagers as predictably pro-parent. When a system is in contention, with members viewing each other as alien, any reaching across the self–other divide can feel to them like a betrayal (Whitaker & Bumberry, 1988, p. 46):

> Overt empathic reflections from the therapist to one particular member of the family can sometimes cut across the task of trying to understand the differences of people's experiences in the family. Particularly in the early stages of the therapeutic work, when family members are not at all sure whether the therapist will be able to appreciate their different struggles, a too overtly understanding response to one person can raise anxiety for other people in the family about your readiness and capacity as a therapist to understand their situations and experiences. (Flaskas, 2009, p. 149)

Many years ago, I held a family session with a 19-year-old, Tasha, and her parents, Kurt and Margaret. After a year of what they all referred to as Tasha's "sobriety," Tasha had, to her parents' dismay, started smoking pot again. Soon after, she lost her job and had a run-in with the law. Tasha and I had been working together since she was 17, mostly individually, and she respected and trusted me. But that didn't prevent her from storming out of the joint meeting with her parents a few minutes into my beginning to engage with her mother empathically. Tasha said in a subsequent individual session that she thought I had been "falling for her shit and taking pity on her." Watching while I made sense of Margaret's disappointment and foreboding, she feared that I was preparing to gang up with her parents against her, and she wasn't about to wait around for that to happen. I lost her and lost the session.

Tasha was wrong about my taking sides. I'd long embraced the Milan Systemic Therapy team's notion of *neutrality* (Selvini Palazzoli et al., 1980)—a commitment to "actively avoid . . . the acceptance of any one position as more correct than another" (Cecchin, 1987, p. 405):

> Neutrality allows us to get away from the tendency of the system to always make definitions and give labels to events. Neutrality takes away labels that define someone as good, bad, sick, healthy, grown up, not grown up, mature, intelligent, et cetera. . . .
>
> Neutrality is to accept the whole system; it's not to be outside or to be cold. It's to feel a sense of compassion, interest, and curiosity about the family's dilemma: How did they get there? How did they organize themselves that way? We try to see the logic. (Cecchin, as cited in Boscolo et al., 1987, pp. 151–152)

Because early readers of the Milan team's work tended to misconstrue neutrality as "the cultivation of a position of *non*involvement" (Cecchin, 1987, p. 405), Kaethe Weingarten suggested *multipartiality* as an alternative term (Sutherland, 2005, p. 8). According to H. Anderson and Goolishian (1988), multipartiality requires a willingness and readiness to entertain "alternative opinions and meanings" by "taking all sides and working with all views simultaneously" (p. 385). This means avoiding

> solicitations or enticements to assume the role of either an adjudicator (judge)—tasked with deciding who's right and who's wrong—or arbitrator—tasked with negotiating a sustainable compromise. . . . Multipartial interaction . . . elicits attention to, validation of, and responsiveness to all . . . points of reference. (Butler et al., 2011, p. 203)

Your commitment to multipartiality is only believable to clients when they see it in action. It isn't enough for you to hold or espouse it as a value; like empathy, multipartiality needs to be shown, not claimed (see Chapter 4). This session and some others like it helped me to fully appreciate why therapeutic conversations sometimes go sideways when the therapist lingers too long, empathically engaging with any one person: Such a focus can be perceived by the other(s) not as evidence of care but of bias.

Multipartiality is easier to demonstrate if you frequently move back and forth between clients, refracting each client's feelings, meanings, motivations, and choices and bringing forth the logic of the interactions between them. You make empathic sense of both intrapersonal experiences and interpersonal patterns of relationship by developing a multifaceted, interwoven acknowledgment of each and everyone in the room—the parts *and* the whole (cf. Stierlin, as cited in Selvini Palazzoli et al., 1978, p. ix; Phelps-Thiry, 1996).

If I were to be granted the opportunity for a redo in the appointment with Tasha and her parents, allowing me to start over from scratch, I'd identify pivot points in the turn-taking that would allow me to move more frequently back and forth between the clients, making it possible for the conversation to unfold in something like the following way.

MARGARET: Tasha thinks of marijuana as medicine,[5] which she prefers to the real medicine the psychiatrist prescribed.

DOUGLAS: As a way of treating her anxiety.

MARGARET: Yes.

Margaret's "yes" puts us in agreement and returns the floor to me, which I use to pivot to her son.

DOUGLAS: Tasha, is your mom right? You use pot as a medication?

TASHA: It calms me down better than any pills.

Tasha and her mom are arguing over the correct classification of marijuana, over its legitimacy. Is it a drug she's using or a medication she's dosing?

MARGARET: But I don't think it works. Now that she's back using, she's on edge, so prickly.

Before attending to Margaret's concern, I acknowledge Tasha's experience, classifying marijuana the way she does:

DOUGLAS: [*to Tasha*] You can feel the immediate, medicinal benefit.

TASHA: Totally.

Her agreement confirms my understanding and returns the floor to me, which I use to now turn back to her mother, this time classifying marijuana in a way that fits for her.

DOUGLAS: [*to Margaret*] But you're worried that the side effects of the drug undermine whatever benefits it offers.

MARGARET: [*nods*]

With both mother and daughter in agreement with me, I'm able to float a statement that holds their contradictory beliefs in juxtaposition without

---

[5] I saw this family several years before medical marijuana was legalized anywhere in the country.

attempting to establish one or the other as true: It isn't a question of whether marijuana helps *or* exacerbates Tasha's anxiety; it helps *and* exacerbates it.

DOUGLAS: [*looks to Tasha*] Tasha, you can tell it calms you down [*pauses and waits for confirmation; she nods*], and [*looks back to Margaret*] you recognize that it puts her on edge.

MARGARET: Yes.

With Margaret accepting my F. Scott Fitzgerald assertion, the time feels right to float an empathic hunch:

DOUGLAS: Which I imagine puts you on edge.

MARGARET: [*nods*]

In the original conversation, Kurt never spoke up or initiated a thought, concern, or opinion. He wasn't checked out; he always responded when I directed a question or empathic comment his way. However, he was inclined to adopt a position as more of a bystander than a participant. In my imagined redo, I more frequently pivot to him.

DOUGLAS: [*turns to Kurt*] What have you been noticing?

KURT: I get why she thinks she needs it.

DOUGLAS: You, too, can see it calming her down?

KURT: In the moment, yes.

DOUGLAS: In the moment. [*turns to Tasha*]

You get the idea. Interlaced empathic refractions and the feedback responses they invite from clients establish a network of mini-connections with everyone involved in the conversation. They allow you to bookmark this interchange with this person at a moment of convergence, with your acknowledging the client's description and/or sensibility and the client's acknowledging that they've been understood. When you then pivot, turning your attention to someone else, the client, feeling heard and respected, can be less concerned that some other person in the room, some nemesis, is going to win your allegiance against them.

> Just when emotions are strongest . . . it is most difficult to achieve the frame of reference of the other person or group. . . . [However,] when the parties in a dispute realize that they are being understood, that someone sees how the situation seems to them, the statements grow less exaggerated and less defensive, and it is no longer necessary to maintain the attitude, "I am 100% right and you are 100% wrong." (Rogers & Roethlisberger, 1952, p. 48)

If you'd like to practice both–and empathizing before bringing it into the therapy room, consider test-driving it at your next big family holiday dinner or at a party where three or four of you are clustered in conversation. Such settings will give you a chance to get a feel for the rhythm of it. Float an empathic comment in response to something one person says. If they take issue with what you offer, try again, correcting or fine-tuning your refraction or hunch until they agree with you. This will return the floor to you, giving you the opportunity to pivot to someone else, smoothing the segue by referencing something the last person said (e.g., "Do you agree with her?" or "I would imagine your take is pretty different").

You probably won't be able to sustain this manner of active interlacing for too long without someone wondering, perhaps aloud, why you've taken it on yourself to host, rather than just participate in, the conversation. Fair. You can keep from drawing undue attention to your practicing both–and refractions by only intermittently sprinkling them throughout casual conversations.

EPILOGUE
Circling Back and Heading Out

I'll stay till the wind changes.
—Mary Poppins, in P. L. Travers's *Mary Poppins* (1934/2014, p. 24)

Let's end by returning to the beginning, to the story of my colleague Sebastian's well-meaning attempt to empathically connect with his client, Nathan. You may recall that in response to Nathan's grousing about his son's decision to move across the country for college, Sebastian had offered an Irvin Yalom–inspired story about his own teeth-gnashing when his daughter had made a similar choice. Nathan was about as receptive to Sebastian's self-disclosure as Cody had been to Randall's (see Chapter 4). So what gives? If Irvin Yalom (2002) had been Nathan or Cody's therapist, would either of them have dismissed him as unceremoniously as they did Sebastian and Randall? Not Nathan, I think, at least not if he knew of Yalom's stature in the field. I suspect he would have looked up to him, as he had his now-deceased older friend and colleague. The status differential would have established a complementary relationship between them, which would have altered how

Nathan received the personal story—more as a gift to be pondered than a mistake to be faulted. Yalom's status might even have been enough to soften Nathan's reaction to a claim of understanding—"If someone as renowned as Dr. Yalom says he knows me," Nathan might have thought, "then perhaps he does." (Yalom's reputation would not have impressed Cody, who was too young and uninformed for it to register, but Yalom's age and bearing might have had some positive influence.) Given that Sebastian couldn't rely on a fame-based free pass, he would have fared much better if he had, as I noted in Chapter 4, demonstrated, rather than claimed, his empathic grasp of Nathan's experience.

The personal story that Sebastian told proposed to Nathan a relationship of *mutual vulnerability* ("I, like you, was hurt by my college-bound senior's bid for distance and freedom"), a proposal that Nathan immediately smacked down. Mutuality-inspired intimacy is sought in friendships but is fraught in clinical settings. It is far better to maintain a complementary relationship that asymmetrically makes it safe for the client to be vulnerable, while allowing the therapist to remain *available*. Such professional intimacy will be easier to pull off if, leaving your ego at the office door (see Figure 2.1), you approach empathic clinical encounters as a mindful practice of untethered, self-less imagining.

You may recall that Sebastian had given Nathan an unvoiced moniker. When the client's name appeared on Sebastian's schedule, he'd mentally prepare for an anticipated tough session by saying to himself, "Okay, gotta gear up for the Bully today." Nathan was overbearing and could be mean, even abusive, at times. It is clear that he intimidated not just his students and colleagues but also his therapist, so it makes sense that Sebastian felt the need for some insulation and protection. His private label for Nathan, like any other form of judging, supplied it. The othering of others diminishes and distances them, rendering them less threatening. I imagine that Sebastian would have considered such judging to be even more necessary after his empathic offering had engendered such a withering, condescending retort: "Am I paying *you* for this session," Nathan had asked, "or are you paying *me*?" (Ouch. Just writing down his statement makes me cringe.)

Remember what I said earlier in this chapter about the importance of interpersonal error correction? I was referring primarily to clients telling us when our empathic hunches are off the mark, but the principle applies just as much to other, more significant missteps. Critical feedback is important in guiding us in getting back in sync with them. I suspect Nathan wouldn't have been amenable to a do-over right after what he considered a professional faux pas, but let's imagine what a follow-up conversation might have looked like if, in the intervening week, Sebastian had done a crash course on what I've covered in this book.

SEBASTIAN: You cut short the session last time. Were you as pissed as you sounded?

Instead of presuming to know what Nathan was feeling, Sebastian ventures to ask. And, in keeping with a lesson I learned from Jacqueline, he inquires about anger, not hurt, a much more comfortable emotion category (Barrett, 2017b) for Nathan to acknowledge. Moreover, he asks about Nathan's (possible) anger toward *him*. The therapeutic alliance needs to be addressed and hopefully repaired before they can move to Nathan's relationship with his son.

NATHAN: As my students will tell you, I don't suffer fools.

Another dig. It would be understandable if Sebastian felt the need to defend himself, but that didn't go well the first time around, so, rather than justify what he did, he's best off empathizing:

SEBASTIAN: Or suffer therapists who share personal details.

By nondefensively making Nathan's insult explicit, Sebastian demonstrates that he is speaking not as a vis-à-vis, but from inside Nathan's world.

NATHAN: You forgot for a moment who was paying whom. Trust me, you can't afford me—my hourly rate is much, much higher than yours.

"You forgot for a moment" signals that Nathan is treating Sebastian's self-disclosure as a glitch, not a pervasive defect. Perhaps Sebastian's nondefensiveness made it possible for Nathan to deliver his almost humorous admonishment in a friendly rather than a demeaning way. Sebastian responds with another empathic statement that bridges into a discussion of Nathan's son.

SEBASTIAN: Besides, you've already got a job or two—teaching, writing [*pauses*]. Three jobs if you count parenting.

NATHAN: I don't get paid for that one.

SEBASTIAN: Even though I imagine that at times it's the hardest.

This hunch gently broaches the issue of Nathan's pain.

NATHAN: At least my students and readers show some appreciation.

SEBASTIAN: Damn kid. Ingrate.

Sebastian is expressing an empathic, not objective, truth: He nonjudgmentally gives voice to what he imagines Nathan's judgment of his son to be. Nathan indirectly agrees.

NATHAN: Idiot.

SEBASTIAN: Choosing some third-rate diploma mill over Harvard? Go figure.

Nathan's son had decided, you may remember, to attend Stanford. Sebastian's characterization meets with appreciation.

NATHAN: [*laughs*] Exactly.

There's nothing like a little humor to relax the self–other boundary. Sharing a laugh helps create a sense of *us*. And Sebastian uses the occasion of Nathan agreeing with him to shift direction.

SEBASTIAN: I got the sense last week that you take his Stanford decision not only as a bone-headed move but also as a middle-finger goodbye.

Nathan doesn't directly agree, but he reveals something he hadn't previously mentioned. Such vulnerability doesn't happen without trust.

NATHAN: He'd told me Stanford was his safety school. He played me.

Sebastian refracts a father's self-recrimination into a compliment about the son.

SEBASTIAN: Played *you*?! At 17? Wow, talk about finesse. No wonder he got into Harvard *and* Stanford.

And his incredulity ("Played *you*?!") also refracts Nathan's sophistication and intelligence, making it more likely that the client will respond magnanimously.

NATHAN: Gotta give him credit.

When a father can be proud of his son besting him, he's not so threatened.

SEBASTIAN: Where's that leave you?

They've arrived at a starting point.

LEAVE-TAKING: EMPATHIC DISENGAGEMENT

As an undertaking and an engagement, empathy is a curiosity-fueled act of imagination-sparked inference. You are guided by what the client describes and displays in conversation with you, as well as by their ongoing corrections of your first, second, third impressions. The client's contributions allow you to begin formulating an impression of how they construct their world—what they're up against, what they're capable of, where they fear they're headed, where they hope to arrive, what they've done to try to get there, who's with and against them, what they're choosing and doing, and so on. In the details they share and you refract, it is possible to identify points of significance (some explicit, others implicit) that, when considered in some kind of constellation, give you both an impression of coherence. Things make sense. Such coherence is a collaborative work of creative nonfiction.

Because the client grants you the privilege of joining them in empathically sketching out and making sense of their world, your trim-tab refractions can become seamlessly incorporated in an updated draft of their story—one that isn't prematurely closed off, one that doesn't yet have a next chapter, one where uncertainty is a feature, not a fear. This is what the client takes with them when they leave.

Leave-taking is a valued part of the client's story, ideally because this new draft sketches you as someone they no longer need. In leaving, the client takes with them the learning they derived from their time with you, learning that shows up and shows through in the way they're now orienting and responding to life's challenges and possibilities.

Leave-taking is also a valued part of reading a book. As you close the cover (or the e-reader app), I hope the learning you've derived from hanging out with me will show up in how you orient and respond to the challenges and possibilities of empathically and therapeutically engaging with your clients. Going forward, the continued development of your conversational artistry (H. Anderson & Goolishian, 1992) will best be developed, refined, and kept fresh by staying continually curious about, and open and responsive to, your clients' feedback (S. D. Miller et al., 2020). Clients are our best teachers. By listening carefully to what they have to offer, you can continue empathically learning *from* them about how to learn empathically *about* them.

References

Alda, A. (Host). (2021, May 3). The empathy diaries with Sherry Turkle [Audio podcast episode]. In *Clear + vivid with Alan Alda*. Apple Podcasts. https://www.sherryturkle.com/post/clear-vivid-with-alan-alda

Anderson, H. (1997). *Conversation, language, and possibilities*. Basic Books.

Anderson, H. (2001). Postmodern collaborative and person-centred therapies: What would Carl Rogers say? *Journal of Family Therapy, 23*(4), 339–360. https://doi.org/10.1111/1467-6427.00189

Anderson, H., & Goolishian, H. A. (1988). Human systems as linguistic systems: Preliminary and evolving ideas about the implications for clinical theory. *Family Process, 27*(4), 371–393. https://doi.org/10.1111/j.1545-5300.1988.00371.x

Anderson, H., & Goolishian, H. A. (1992). The client is the expert: A not-knowing approach to therapy. In S. McNamee & K. J. Gergen (Eds.), *Therapy as social construction* (pp. 25–39). Sage.

Anderson, R., & Cissna, K. N. (1997). *The Martin Buber–Carl Rogers dialogue: A new transcript with commentary*. State University of New York Press.

Aragno, A. (2008). The language of empathy: An analysis of its constitution, development, and role in psychoanalytic listening. *Journal of the American Psychoanalytic Association, 56*(3), 713–740. https://doi.org/10.1177/0003065108322097

Armstrong, J. (Executive Producer). (2018–2023). *Succession* [TV series]. HBO Entertainment; Gary Sanchez Productions; Hyperobject Industries; Hot Seat Productions; Project Zeus.

Arnold, K. (2014). Behind the mirror: Reflective listening and its tain in the work of Carl Rogers. *The Humanistic Psychologist, 42*(4), 354–369. https://doi.org/10.1080/08873267.2014.913247

Aylward, M. (2021). *Awake where you are: The art of embodied awareness*. Wisdom Publications.

Baldwin, M. (1987). Interview with Carl Rogers on the use of the self in therapy. In M. Baldwin & V. Satir (Eds.), *The use of self in therapy* (pp. 29–38). Routledge.

Barrett, L. F. (2017a). *How emotions are made: The secret life of the brain*. HarperCollins.

Barrett, L. F. (2017b). The theory of constructed emotion: An active inference account of interoception and categorization. *Social Cognitive and Affective Neuroscience, 12*(11), 1–23. Advance online publication. https://doi.org/10.1093/scan/nsx060

Barrett, L. F. (2020). *Seven and a half lessons about the brain*. Houghton Mifflin Harcourt.

Barrett, L. F., & Quigley, K. S. (2021, July 1). Interoception: The secret ingredient. *Cerebrum*. https://www.ncbi.nlm.nih.gov/pmc/articles/PMC8493823/pdf/cer-06-21.pdf

Barrett, L. F., Quigley, K. S., & Hamilton, P. (2016). An active inference theory of allostasis and interoception in depression. *Philosophical Transactions of the Royal Society of London B: Biological Sciences, 371*(1708), Article 20160011. https://doi.org/10.1098/rstb.2016.0011

Barrett, L. F., & Russell, J. A. (1998). Independence and bipolarity in the structure of current affect. *Journal of Personality and Social Psychology, 74*(4), 967–984. https://doi.org/10.1037/0022-3514.74.4.967

Basch, M. F. (1983). Empathic understanding: A review of the concept and some theoretical considerations. *Journal of the American Psychoanalytic Association, 31*(1), 101–126. https://doi.org/10.1177/000306518303100104

Basch, M. F. (1990). Further thoughts on empathic understanding. In A. Goldberg (Ed.), *The realities of transference* (pp. 3–10). Analytic Press.

Batchelor, S. (1997). *Buddhism without beliefs*. Riverhead Books.

Bateson, G. (with Bateson, M. C.). (2000). *Steps to an ecology of mind*. The University of Chicago Press. (Original work published 1972)

Bateson, G. (2002). *Mind and nature: A necessary unity*. Hampton Press. (Original work published 1979)

Bateson, G., & Bateson, M. C. (1987). *Angels fear: Towards an epistemology of the sacred*. Macmillan.

Batson, C. D. (2009). These things called empathy: Eight related but distinct phenomena. In J. Decety & W. Ickes (Eds.), *The social neuroscience of empathy* (pp. 3–16). MIT Press. https://doi.org/10.7551/mitpress/9780262012973.003.0002

Batson, C. D. (2023). *Empathic concern: What it is and why it's important*. Oxford University Press. https://doi.org/10.1093/oso/9780197610923.001.0001

Batson, C. D., Early, S., & Salvarani, G. (1997). Perspective taking: Imagining how another feels versus imagining how you would feel. *Personality and Social Psychology Bulletin, 23*(7), 751–758. https://doi.org/10.1177/0146167297237008

Bavelas, J. B., Coates, L., & Johnson, T. (2000). Listeners as co-narrators. *Journal of Personality and Social Psychology, 79*(6), 941–952. https://doi.org/10.1037/0022-3514.79.6.941

Becvar, D. S., & Becvar, R. J. (2013). *Family therapy: A systemic integration* (8th ed.). Pearson.

Bergen, B. K. (2013). Metaphors are in the mind. In J. Brockman (Ed.), *This explains everything* (pp. 218–220). Harper Perennial.

Berlin, I. (1976). *Vico and Herder: Two studies in the history of ideas*. Vintage Books.

Bernhardt, B. C., & Singer, T. (2012). The neural basis of empathy. *Annual Review of Neuroscience, 35*(1), 1–23. https://doi.org/10.1146/annurev-neuro-062111-150536

Besman-Albinder, S. (2006). *The impact of trauma work on resilient therapists and their partners* [Unpublished doctoral dissertation]. Nova Southeastern University.

Blake, W. (ca. 1803). *The grey monk* [Manuscript]. The Morgan Library & Museum. https://www.themorgan.org/sites/default/files/pdf/facsimile/BlakeMA2879.pdf

Bloom, P. (2016). *Against empathy: The case for rational compassion*. HarperCollins.

Bloom, P., & Zaki, J. (2016, December 29). Does empathy guide or hinder moral action? *The New York Times*. https://www.nytimes.com/roomfordebate/2016/12/29/does-empathy-guide-or-hinder-moral-action

Bochner, A. (2014). *Coming to narrative*. Left Coast Press.

Bohart, A. C., & Greenberg, L. S. (1997a). Empathy and psychotherapy: An introductory overview. In A. C. Bohart & L. S. Greenberg (Eds.), *Empathy reconsidered: New directions in psychotherapy* (pp. 3–31). American Psychological Association. https://doi.org/10.1037/10226-018

Bohart, A. C., & Greenberg, L. S. (1997b). Empathy: Where are we and where do we go from here? In A. C. Bohart & L. S. Greenberg (Eds.), *Empathy reconsidered: New directions in psychotherapy* (pp. 419–449). American Psychological Association. https://doi.org/10.1037/10226-031

Bohart, A. C., & Rosenbaum, R. (1995). The dance of empathy: Empathy, diversity, and technical eclecticism. *The Person-Centered Journal, 2*(1), 5–29. https://www.adpca.org/wp-content/uploads/2020/11/V2-N1-4.pdf

Borke, H. (1971). Interpersonal perception of young children: Egocentrism or empathy? *Developmental Psychology, 5*(2), 263–269. https://doi.org/10.1037/h0031267

Boscolo, L., Cecchin, G., Hoffman, L., & Penn, P. (1987). *Milan systemic family therapy: Conversations in theory and practice*. Basic Books.

Bowen, L. (Writer), & Lowney, D. (Director). (2020, September 18). The diamond dogs (Season 1, Episode 8) [TV series episode]. In B. Lawrence, J. Sudeikis, J. Ingold, & B. Wrubel (Executive Producers), *Ted Lasso*. Apple TV; Ruby's Tuna; Universal Television; Doozer; Warner Bros. Television.

Bozarth, J. D. (1997). Empathy from the framework of client-centered theory and the Rogerian hypothesis. In A. C. Bohart & L. S. Greenberg (Eds.), *Empathy reconsidered: New directions in psychotherapy* (pp. 81–102). American Psychological Association. https://doi.org/10.1037/10226-003

Bozarth, J. D. (2009). Rogerian empathy in an organismic theory: A way of being. In J. Decety & W. Ickes (Eds.), *The social neuroscience of empathy* (pp. 101–112). MIT Press.

Bridges, J., & Glassman, B. (2012). *The Dude and the Zen master*. Blue Rider Press.

Briere, J. (2012). Working with trauma: Mindfulness and compassion. In R. D. Siegel & C. K. Germer (Eds.), *Wisdom and compassion in psychotherapy* (pp. 265–279). Guilford Press.

Brooks, D. (2023). *How to know a person*. Random House.

Brown, B. (2018). *Dare to lead*. Random House.

Brown, K. W., & Ryan, R. M. (2003). The benefits of being present: Mindfulness and its role in psychological well-being. *Journal of Personality and Social Psychology, 84*(4), 822–848. https://doi.org/10.1037/0022-3514.84.4.822

Buber, M. (1970). *I and thou: A new translation with a prologue and notes by Walter Kaufmann* (W. Kaufmann, Trans.). Scribner. (Original work published 1923)

Butler, M. H., Brimhall, A. S., & Harper, J. M. (2011). A primer on the evolution of therapeutic engagement in MFT: Understanding and resolving the dialectic tension of alliance and neutrality. Part 2—Recommendations: Dynamic neutrality through multipartiality and enactments. *The American Journal of Family Therapy, 39*(3), 193–213. https://doi.org/10.1080/01926187.2010.493112

Cadge, W., & Hammonds, C. (2012). Reconsidering detached concern: The case of intensive-care nurses. *Perspectives in Biology and Medicine, 55*(2), 266–282. https://doi.org/10.1353/pbm.2012.0021

Cairns, P., Isham, A. E., & Zachariae, R. (2024). The association between empathy and burnout in medical students: A systematic review and meta-analysis. *BMC Medical Education, 24*(1), 640. https://doi.org/10.1186/s12909-024-05625-6

Carraça, B., Serpa, S., Palmi, J., & Rosado, A. (2018). Enhance sport performance of elite athletes: The mindfulness-based interventions. *Cuadernos de Psicología del Deporte, 18*(2), 79–109. https://psycnet.apa.org/record/2018-30930-007

Carroll, L. (2009). *Alice's adventures in Wonderland and through the looking glass*. Digireads.com (Original work published 1872)

Carson, J. (1991). What I have learned. *Johnny Carson Tonight Show script collection* (No. 2630, Box 22, Folders 56 & 57). Online Archive of California. https://oac.cdlib.org/findaid/ark:/13030/c8rf5wpf/entire_text/

Cecchin, G. (1987). Hypothesizing, circularity, and neutrality revisited: An invitation to curiosity. *Family Process, 26*(4), 405–413. https://doi.org/10.1111/j.1545-5300.1987.00405.x

Chan, Z. C., Fung, Y., & Chien, W. (2013). Bracketing in phenomenology: Only undertaken in the data collection and analysis process? *The Qualitative Report, 18*(30), 1–9. https://doi.org/10.46743/2160-3715/2013.1486

Chen, H., Xuan, H., Cai, J., Liu, M., & Shi, L. (2024). The impact of empathy on medical students: An integrative review. *BMC Medical Education, 24*(1), 455. https://doi.org/10.1186/s12909-024-05448-5

Chödrön, P. (2001). *The places that scare you*. Shambhala.

Chödrön, P. (2013). *How to meditate*. Sounds True.

Chödrön, P. (2016). *When things fall apart*. Shambhala.

Cissna, K. N., & Anderson, R. (2002). *Moments of meeting: Buber, Rogers, and the potential for public dialogue*. State University of New York Press.

Clark, A. J. (2007). *Empathy in counseling and psychotherapy*. Routledge.

Clark, A. J. (2010). Empathy and sympathy: Therapeutic distinctions in counseling. *Journal of Mental Health Counseling, 32*(2), 95–101. https://doi.org/10.17744/mehc.32.2.228n116thw397504

Cohen, T. (1999). Identifying with metaphor: Metaphors of personal identification. *The Journal of Aesthetics and Art Criticism, 57*(4), 399–409. https://doi.org/10.2307/432147

Cohen, T. (2008). *Thinking of others: On the talent for metaphor*. Princeton University Press.

Colbert, S. (Host). (2022, November 11). Author George Saunders [Audio Podcast Episode]. In *The Late Show Pod Show with Stephen Colbert*. CBS.

Colvin, S. (Ed.). (2011). *Letters of John Keats to his family and friends*. Project Gutenberg. https://www.gutenberg.org/files/35698/35698-h/35698-h.htm (Original work published 1891)

Coplan, A. (2011a). Understanding empathy: Its features and effects. In A. Coplan & P. Goldie (Eds.), *Empathy: Philosophical and psychological perspectives* (pp. 3–18). Oxford University Press.

Coplan, A. (2011b). Will the real empathy please stand up? A case for a narrow conceptualization [Special issue]. *The Southern Journal of Philosophy, 49*(s1), 40–65. https://doi.org/10.1111/j.2041-6962.2011.00056.x

Crichton, M. (2008). *Prey*. Harper.

Crumlin, J. (2021, May 19). *Intense acting roles: Immersion and sustainability*. StageMilk. https://www.stagemilk.com/intense-acting-roles/

Csikszentmihalyi, M. (1990). *Flow: The psychology of optimal experience*. Harper Perennial.

Cuff, B. M. P., Brown, S. J., Taylor, L., & Howat, D. J. (2016). Empathy: A review of the concept. *Emotion Review, 8*(2), 144–153. https://doi.org/10.1177/1754073914558466

Davidson, R. J., & Harrington, A. (2002). Dialogues, part II: Pragmatic extensions and applications. In R. J. Davidson & A. Harrison (Eds.), *Visions of compassion: Western scientists and Tibetan Buddhists examine human nature* (pp. 213–246). Oxford University Press.

Davies, C. (2024, August 15). *The Crown's* Elizabeth Debicki says she struggled to leave Diana's mannerisms behind. *The Guardian*. https://www.theguardian.com/tv-and-radio/article/2024/aug/15/the-crowns-elizabeth-debicki-says-she-struggled-to-leave-mannerisms-of-princess-diana-behind

Davis, B. B. (2021). *Self, other, and empathy in relational supervision: An IPR investigation* (Publication No. 28770322) [Doctoral dissertation, Nova Southeastern University]. ProQuest Dissertations and Theses Global.

Davis, M. H. (2017). Empathy in twentieth-century psychology. In H. L. Maibom (Ed.), *The Routledge handbook of philosophy of empathy* (pp. 110–121). Taylor & Francis.

Davis, M. H., Hull, J. G., Young, R. D., & Warren, G. G. (1987). Emotional reactions to dramatic film stimuli: The influence of cognitive and emotional empathy.

Journal of Personality and Social Psychology, *52*(1), 126–133. https://doi.org/10.1037/0022-3514.52.1.126

Debes, R. (2017). Empathy and mirror neurons. In H. L. Maibom (Ed.), *The Routledge handbook of philosophy of empathy* (pp. 54–63). Taylor & Francis.

Decety, J., & Jackson, P. L. (2004). The functional architecture of human empathy. *Behavioral and Cognitive Neuroscience Reviews*, *3*(2), 71–100. https://doi.org/10.1177/1534582304267187

Decety, J., & Lamm, C. (2009). Empathy versus personal distress: Recent evidence from social neuroscience. In J. Decety & W. Ickes (Eds.), *The social neuroscience of empathy* (pp. 199–212). MIT Press.

Delgado, N., Delgado, J., Betancort, M., Bonache, H., & Harris, L. T. (2023). What is the link between different components of empathy and burnout in healthcare professionals? A systematic review and meta-analysis. *Psychology Research and Behavior Management*, *16*, 447–463. https://doi.org/10.2147/PRBM.S384247

de Saussure, F. (1987). *Course in general linguistics* (P. Meisel & H. Saussy, Eds.; W. Baskin, Trans.). Columbia University Press. (Original work published 1916)

Descartes, R. (1911). *The philosophical works of Descartes* (E. S. Haldane & G. R. T. Ross, Trans.). Cambridge University Press. (Original work published 1641)

de Vignemont, F., & Singer, T. (2006). The empathic brain: How, when and why? *Trends in Cognitive Sciences*, *10*(10), 435–441. https://doi.org/10.1016/j.tics.2006.08.008

di Pellegrino, G., Fadiga, L., Fogassi, L., Gallese, V., & Rizzolatti, G. (1992). Understanding motor events: A neurophysiological study. *Experimental Brain Research*, *91*(1), 176–180. https://doi.org/10.1007/BF00230027

Dowd, M. (2022, October 22). Ralph Fiennes, master of monsters. *The New York Times*. https://www.nytimes.com/2022/10/22/style/ralph-fiennes-robert-moses.html

Duncan, S., & Barrett, L. F. (2007). Affect is a form of cognition: A neurobiological analysis. *Cognition and Emotion*, *21*(6), 1184–1211. https://doi.org/10.1080/02699930701437931

Dunning, D. (2011). The Dunning–Kruger effect: On being ignorant of one's own ignorance. In J. M. Olson & M. P. Zanna (Eds.), *Advances in experimental social psychology* (Vol. 44, pp. 247–296). Academic Press. https://doi.org/10.1016/B978-0-12-385522-0.00005-6

Duradoni, M., Gursesli, M. C., Fiorenza, M., Donati, A., & Guazzini, A. (2023). Cognitive empathy and the dark triad: A literature review. *European Journal of Investigation in Health, Psychology and Education*, *13*(11), 2642–2680. https://doi.org/10.3390/ejihpe13110184

Durrell, L. (1957). *The Alexandria quartet*. E. P. Dutton.

Dymond, R. F. (1949). A scale for the measurement of empathic ability. *Journal of Consulting Psychology*, *13*(2), 127–133. https://doi.org/10.1037/h0061728

Edwards, L. H. (2013). A brief conceptual history of Einfühlung: 18th-century Germany to post-World War II U.S. psychology. *History of Psychology*, *16*(4), 269–281. https://doi.org/10.1037/a0033634

Egan, G., & Reese, R. J. (2019). *The skilled helper* (11th ed.). Cengage.
Eisenberg, N., & Eggum, N. D. (2009). Empathic responding: Sympathy and personal distress. In J. Decety & W. Ickes (Eds.), *The social neuroscience of empathy* (pp. 71–83). MIT Press.
Eisenberg, N., Shea, C. L., Carlo, G., & Knight, G. (1991). Empathy-related responding and cognition: A "chicken and the egg" dilemma. In W. Kurtines & J. Gewirtz (Eds.), *Handbook of moral behavior and development: Vol. 2. Research* (pp. 63–88). Erlbaum.
Eisenberg, N., & Strayer, J. (1987). Critical issues in the study of empathy. In N. Eisenberg & J. Strayer (Eds.), *Empathy and its development* (pp. 3–13). Cambridge University Press.
Ekman, P. (Ed.). (2021). *Emotion in the human face*. Malor Books.
Ekman, P., & Cordaro, D. (2011). What is meant by calling emotions basic. *Emotion Review*, *3*(4), 364–370. https://doi.org/10.1177/1754073911410740
Elliott, R., Bohart, A. C., Watson, J. C., & Greenberg, L. S. (2011). Empathy. *Psychotherapy*, *48*(1), 43–49. https://doi.org/10.1037/a0022187
Elliott, R., Bohart, A. C., Watson, J. C., & Murphy, D. (2018). Therapist empathy and client outcome: An updated meta-analysis. *Psychotherapy*, *55*(4), 399–410. https://doi.org/10.1037/pst0000175
Epstein, M. (1995). *Thoughts without a thinker*. Basic Books.
Epstein, R. (2017). *Attending: Medicine, mindfulness, and humanity*. Scribner.
Erickson, M. H. (2008a). Further clinical techniques of hypnosis: Utilization techniques. In E. L. Rossi, R. Erickson-Klein, & K. L. Rossi (Eds.), *The collected works of Milton H. Erickson* (Vol. 1, pp. 271–301). The Milton H. Erickson Foundation Press.
Erickson, M. H. (2008b). Hypnosis: Its renascence as a treatment modality. In E. L. Rossi, R. Erickson-Klein, & K. L. Rossi (Eds.), *The collected works of Milton H. Erickson* (Vol. 2, pp. 61–85). The Milton H. Erickson Foundation Press.
Erickson, M. H., & Rossi, E. L. (2014). The indirect forms of suggestion. In E. L. Rossi, R. Erickson-Klein, & K. L. Rossi (Eds.), *The collected works of Milton H. Erickson* (Vol. 11, pp. 18–52). The Milton H. Erickson Foundation Press.
Erickson, M. H., & Zeig, J. (2008). Symptom prescription for expanding the psychotic's world view. In E. L. Rossi, R. Erickson-Klein, & K. L. Rossi (Eds.), *The collected works of Milton H. Erickson* (Vol. 4, pp. 285–288). The Milton H. Erickson Foundation Press.
Evon, D. (2021, August 5). *Did "be curious, not judgmental" originate with Walt Whitman?* Snopes. https://www.snopes.com/fact-check/be-curious-not-judgmental-walt-whitman/
Eyal, T., Steffel, M., & Epley, N. (2018). Perspective mistaking: Accurately understanding the mind of another requires getting perspective, not taking perspective. *Journal of Personality and Social Psychology*, *114*(4), 547–571. https://doi.org/10.1037/pspa0000115
Feagan, S. L. (2011). Empathizing as simulating. In A. Coplan & P. Goldie (Eds.), *Empathy: Philosophical and psychological perspectives* (pp. 149–161). Oxford University Press.

Feldman, C., & Kuyken, W. (2011). Compassion in the landscape of suffering. *Contemporary Buddhism*, *12*(1), 143–155. https://doi.org/10.1080/14639947.2011.564831

Figley, C. R. (1995). Compassion fatigue as secondary traumatic stress disorder: An overview. In C. R. Figley (Ed.), *Compassion fatigue: Coping with secondary traumatic stress disorder in those who treat the traumatized* (pp. 1–20). Routledge.

Figley, C. R. (2012). The empathic response in clinical practice: Antecedents and consequences. In J. Decety (Ed.), *Empathy: From bench to bedside* (pp. 263–274). MIT Press.

Firestein, S. (2012). *Ignorance: How it drives science*. Oxford University Press.

Firestein, S. (2016). *Failure: Why science is so successful*. Oxford University Press.

Fischer, N. (2013). *Training in compassion: Zen teachings on the practice of Lojong*. Shambhala.

Fitzgerald, F. S. (1936, February 1). The crack-up. *Esquire*. https://classic.esquire.com/article/share/97a6b0a8-ba1c-4b7b-aa64-0d08dd9fb952

Fitzgerald, F. T. (1999). Curiosity. *Annals of Internal Medicine*, *130*(1), 70–72. https://doi.org/10.7326/0003-4819-130-1-199901050-00015

Flaskas, C. (2009). The therapist's imagination of self in relation to clients: Beginning ideas on the flexibility of empathic imagination. *Australian and New Zealand Journal of Family Therapy*, *30*(3), 147–159. https://doi.org/10.1375/anft.30.3.147

Flaskas, C. (2018). What would (or can) I know? Reflections on the conditions of knowing and understanding in intercultural therapy. In I. Krause (Ed.), *Culture and reflexivity in systemic psychotherapy: Mutual perspectives* (pp. 53–70). Routledge.

Fleischacker, S. (2019). *Being me being you: Adam Smith and empathy*. University of Chicago Press.

Flemons, D. (1991). *Completing distinctions: Interweaving the ideas of Gregory Bateson and Taoism into a unique approach to therapy*. Shambhala.

Flemons, D. (2002). *Of one mind: The logic of hypnosis, the practice of therapy*. Norton.

Flemons, D. (2020). Toward a relational theory of hypnosis. *American Journal of Clinical Hypnosis*, *62*(4), 344–363. https://doi.org/10.1080/00029157.2019.1666700

Flemons, D. (with Yapko, M. D.). (2022). *The heart and mind of hypnotherapy: Inviting connection, inventing change*. Norton.

Flemons, D., & Gralnik, L. M. (with Meichenbaum, D.). (2013). *Relational suicide assessment: Risks, resources, and possibilities for safety*. Norton.

Flemons, D., & Green, S. (2018). Therapeutic quickies: Brief relational therapy for sexual issues. In S. Green & D. Flemons (Eds.), *Quickies: The handbook of brief sex therapy* (3rd ed., pp. 9–45). Norton.

Fliess, R. (1942). The metapsychology of the analyst. *The Psychoanalytic Quarterly*, *11*(2), 211–227. https://doi.org/10.1080/21674086.1942.11925496

Flückiger, C., Del Re, A. C., Wampold, B. E., & Horvath, A. O. (2018). The alliance in adult psychotherapy: A meta-analytic synthesis. *Psychotherapy*, *55*(4), 316–340.

Fragoso, S. (Host). (2023, October 15). A human conversation with writer George Saunders [Audio podcast episode]. In *Talk Easy*. https://talkeasypod.com/play-it-again-george-saunders/

Fragoso, S. (Host). (2024, August 29). Director Steven Soderbergh: Scene by scene [Audio podcast episode]. In *Talk Easy*. https://talkeasypod.com/play-it-again-steven-soderbergh/

Frankel, R. M. (2017). The evolution of empathy research: Models, muddles, and mechanisms. *Patient Education and Counseling*, *100*(11), 2128–2130. https://doi.org/10.1016/j.pec.2017.05.004

Fraser, S. J., & Solovey, A. D. (2007). *Second-order change in psychotherapy: The golden thread that unifies effective treatments*. American Psychological Association. https://doi.org/10.1037/11499-000

Freudenberger, H. J. (1974). Staff burn-out. *Journal of Social Issues*, *30*(1), 159–165. https://doi.org/10.1111/j.1540-4560.1974.tb00706.x

Fridman, L. (Host). (2020, October 4). Lisa Feldman Barrett: Counterintuitive ideas about how the brain works (No. 129) [Audio podcast episode]. In *Lex Fridman Podcast*. Apple Inc. https://podcasts.apple.com/us/podcast/lex-fridmanpodcast/id1434243584?i=1000493544039#129

Friedman, A. (2019). Cultural blind spots and blind fields: Collective forms of unawareness. In W. H. Brekhus & G. Ignatow (Eds.), *The Oxford handbook of cognitive sociology* (pp. 467–482). Oxford University Press. https://doi.org/10.1093/oxfordhb/9780190273385.013.25

Friedman, M. (1986). Carl Rogers and Martin Buber: Self-actualization and dialogue. *Person-Centered Review*, *1*(4), 409–435.

Fronsdal, G. (2003, October 26). *Not knowing mind* [Audio]. Insight Meditation Center. https://www.audiodharma.org/talks/395

FX Networks. (2022, July 13). *Carmy's 7-minute monologue | The Bear | FX* [Video]. YouTube. https://www.youtube.com/watch?v=1fjITOkFnnE

Gardiner, A., Gleeson, S., Heyward, M., LaBonte, B., Porchia, D., Robb, A., Tipoki, P., & Zanotto, D. (n.d.). *Your pocket guide to de-role*. The Arts Wellbeing Collective. https://www.artswellbeingcollective.com.au/resources/your-pocket-guide-to-post-show-de-role/

Gardner, R., Fitzgerald, R., & Mushin, I. (2009). The underlying orderliness in turn-taking: Examples from Australian talk. *Australian Journal of Communication*, *36*(3), 65–89.

Garville, S. (n.d.). *Parting with a part: How to de-role*. Spotlight. https://www.spotlight.com/news-and-advice/the-essentials/parting-with-a-part-how-to-de-role/#:~:text=Some%20actors%20recommend%20showering%20straight,strengthen%20their%20sense%20of%20self

Geller, S. M., & Greenberg, L. S. (2023). *Therapeutic presence: A mindful approach to effective therapeutic relationships* (2nd ed.). American Psychological Association. https://doi.org/10.1037/0000315-000

Gendlin, E. T. (1981). *Focusing*. Bantam Books.

Gendlin, E. T. (1992). Celebrations and problems of humanistic psychology. *The Humanistic Psychologist, 20*(2–3), 447–460. https://doi.org/10.1080/08873267.1992.9986809

Germer, C. K. (2012). Cultivating compassion in psychotherapy. In R. D. Siegel & C. K. Germer (Eds.), *Wisdom and compassion in psychotherapy* (pp. 93–110). Guilford Press.

Gilbert, P., & Choden. (2014). *Mindful compassion*. New Harbinger.

Glatch, S. (2022, December 6). *"Show, don't tell" in creative writing*. Writers.com. https://writers.com/show-dont-tell-writing

Gleichgerrcht, E., & Decety, J. (2012). The costs of empathy among health professionals. In J. Decety (Ed.), *Empathy: From bench to bedside* (pp. 245–262). MIT Press.

Goldie, P. (2011). Anti-empathy. In A. Coplan & P. Goldie (Eds.), *Empathy: Philosophical and psychological perspectives* (pp. 302–317). Oxford University Press.

Goldman, A. I. (2011). Two routes to empathy: Insights from cognitive neuroscience. In A. Coplan & P. Goldie (Eds.), *Empathy: Philosophical and psychological perspectives* (pp. 31–44). Oxford University Press.

Goldman, R. N., Vaz, A., & Rousmaniere, T. (2021). *Deliberate practice in emotion-focused therapy*. American Psychological Association. https://doi.org/10.1037/0000227-000

Goldstein, J. (2002). *One dharma: The emerging Western Buddhism*. HarperCollins.

Goldstein, J. (2016). *Mindfulness: A practical guide to awakening*. Sounds True.

Goldstein, J. (2020). *Essential advice: 2. Dealing with distractions* [Audio meditation]. Happier.

Goodwin, C., & Heritage, J. (1990). Conversation analysis. *Annual Review of Anthropology, 19*(1), 283–307. https://doi.org/10.1146/annurev.an.19.100190.001435

Gordon, M. (1998). *Spending*. Simon & Schuster.

Goubert, L., Craig, K. D., & Buysse, A. (2009). Perceiving others in pain: Experimental and clinical evidence on the role of empathy. In J. Decety & W. Ickes (Eds.), *The social neuroscience of empathy* (pp. 153–165). MIT Press.

Greenberg, L. S., & Elliott, R. (1997). Varieties of empathic responding. In A. C. Bohart & L. S. Greenberg (Eds.), *Empathy reconsidered: New directions in psychotherapy* (pp. 167–186). American Psychological Association. https://doi.org/10.1037/10226-007

Gunaratana, B. H. (2011). *Mindfulness in plain English*. Wisdom Publications.

Gündem, D., Potočnik, J., De Winter, F. L., El Kaddouri, A., Stam, D., Peeters, R., Emsell, L., Sunaert, S., Van Oudenhove, L., Vandenbulcke, M., Feldman Barrett, L., & Van den Stock, J. (2022). The neurobiological basis of affect is consistent with psychological construction theory and shares a common neural basis across emotional categories. *Communications Biology, 5*(1), 1354. Advance online publication. https://doi.org/10.1038/s42003-022-04324-6

Gunnison, H. (1985, May). The uniqueness of similarities: Parallels of Milton H. Erickson and Carl Rogers. *Journal of Counseling and Development, 63*(9), 561–564. https://doi.org/10.1002/j.1556-6676.1985.tb00681.x

Gutsell, J. N., & Inzlicht, M. (2010). Empathy constrained: Prejudice predicts reduced mental simulation of actions during observation of outgroups. *Journal of Experimental Social Psychology, 46*(5), 841–845. https://doi.org/10.1016/j.jesp.2010.03.011

Hagen, S. (2003). *Buddhism is not what you think*. HarperCollins.

Haley, J. (1981). *Reflections on therapy and other essays*. The Family Therapy Institute.

Haley, J. (1986). *Uncommon therapy: The psychiatric techniques of Milton H. Erickson, M.D.* Norton.

Hallenbeck, P. N. (1981). "Empathy: A neglected topic in psychological research": Reply. *American Psychologist, 36*(2), 225–226. https://doi.org/10.1037/0003-066X.36.2.225

Halpern, J. (2001). *From detached concern to empathy: Humanizing medical practice*. Oxford University Press.

Halpern, J. (2012). Clinical empathy in medical care. In J. Decety (Ed.), *Empathy: From bench to bedside* (pp. 229–244). MIT Press.

Harari, E. (1996). Empathy and the therapeutic relationship in systemic-oriented therapies: A historical and clinical overview. In C. Flaskas & A. Perlesz (Eds.), *The therapeutic relationship in systemic therapy* (pp. 53–70). Karnac Books.

Harrington, A. (2002). A science of compassion or a compassionate science? What do we expect from a cross-cultural dialogue with Buddhism? In R. J. Davidson & A. Harrington (Eds.), *Visions of compassion: Western scientists and Tibetan Buddhists examine human nature* (pp. 18–30). Oxford University Press. https://doi.org/10.1093/acprof:oso/9780195130430.003.0002

Harris, D. (2014). *Ten percent happier*. HarperCollins.

Harris, D., & Warren, J. (2017). *Meditation for fidgety skeptics*. Harmony Books.

Harris, S. (2014). *Waking up*. Simon & Schuster.

Hermansson, G. (1997). Boundaries and boundary management in counselling: The never-ending story. *British Journal of Guidance & Counselling, 25*(2), 133–146. https://doi.org/10.1080/03069889708253797

Hill-hain, A., & Rogers, C. R. (1988). A dialogue with Carl Rogers: Cross-cultural challenges of facilitating person-centered groups in South Africa. *Journal for Specialists in Group Work, 13*(2), 62–69. https://doi.org/10.1080/01933928808411777

Hirschberg, L. (2006, January 15). Buttoned up. *The New York Times Magazine*. https://www.nytimes.com/2006/01/15/magazine/buttoned-up.html

Hirshfield, J. (1997). *Nine gates: Entering the mind of poetry*. HarperPerennial.

Hoffman, L. (1993). *Exchanging voices: A collaborative approach to family therapy*. Taylor & Francis.

Hojat, M. (2016). *Empathy in health professions education and patient care*. Springer. https://doi.org/10.1007/978-3-319-27625-0

Hötzel, M. J., Vieira, M. C., & Leme, D. P. (2019). Exploring horse owners' and caretakers' perceptions of emotions and associated behaviors in horses. *Journal of Veterinary Behavior*, *29*, 18–24. https://doi.org/10.1016/j.jveb.2018.10.002

Houshmand, Z., Harrington, A., Saron, C., & Davidson, R. (2002). Training the mind: First steps in a cross-cultural collaboration in neuroscientific research. In R. J. Davidson & A. Harrington (Eds.), *Visions of compassion: Western scientists and Tibetan Buddhists examine human nature* (pp. 3–17). Oxford University Press. https://doi.org/10.1093/acprof:oso/9780195130430.003.0001

Huberman, A. (Host). (2023, October 16). Dr. Lisa Feldman Barrett: How to understand emotions (No. 146) [Audio podcast episode]. In *Huberman Lab*. https://podcasts.apple.com/us/podcast/huberman-lab/id1545953110?i=1000631446646

Hui, J., Cashman, T., & Deacon, T. (2008). Bateson's method: Double description. What is it? How does it work? What do we learn? In J. Hoffmeyer (Ed.), *A legacy for living systems: Gregory Bateson as precursor to biosemiotics* (pp. 77–92). Springer. https://doi.org/10.1007/978-1-4020-6706-8_6

Hume, D. (1739). *A treatise of human nature*.

Ickes, W. (Ed.). (1997). *Empathic accuracy*. Guilford Press.

Ickes, W. (2011). Everyday mind reading is driven by motives and goals. *Psychological Inquiry*, *22*(3), 200–206. https://doi.org/10.1080/1047840X.2011.561133

Ickes, W., Stinson, L., Bissonnette, V., & Garcia, S. (1990). Naturalistic social cognition: Empathic accuracy in mixed-sex dyads. *Journal of Personality and Social Psychology*, *59*(4), 730–742. https://doi.org/10.1037/0022-3514.59.4.730

Imel, Z. E., Barco, J. S., Brown, H. J., Baucom, B. R., Baer, J. S., Kircher, J. C., & Atkins, D. C. (2014). The association of therapist empathy and synchrony in vocally encoded arousal. *Journal of Counseling Psychology*, *61*(1), 146–153. https://doi.org/10.1037/a0034943

Isaacson, W. (2015, October 30). The light-beam rider. *The New York Times*. https://www.nytimes.com/2015/11/01/opinion/sunday/the-light-beam-rider.html

Ivey, A. E. (1971). *Microcounseling*. Charles C. Thomas.

Ivey, A. E., Ivey, M. B., & Zalaquett, C. P. (2010). *Intentional interviewing and counseling* (7th ed.). Brooks Cole.

Jackson, P. (2006). *Sacred hoops*. Hachette Books.

Jahoda, G. (2005, Spring). Theodor Lipps and the shift from "sympathy" to "empathy." *Journal of the History of the Behavioral Sciences*, *41*(2), 151–163. https://doi.org/10.1002/jhbs.20080

Jamison, L. (2014). *The empathy exams*. Graywolf Press.

Jinpa, T. (2015). *A fearless heart*. Hudson Street Press.

Joinson, C. (1992, April). Coping with compassion fatigue. *Nursing, 22*(4), 116–121. https://doi.org/10.1097/00152193-199204000-00035

Jones, T. (2022, October 17). Are there sports stars that use meditation as part of training? *Ungloo.* https://ungloo.com/blogs/meditation/are-there-sports-stars-that-use-meditation-as-part-of-training

Kabat-Zinn, J. (1990). *Full catastrophe living.* Random House.

Kabat-Zinn, J. (2005). *Wherever you go, there you are: Mindfulness meditation in everyday life.* Hyperion.

Kabat-Zinn, J. (2023). *Mindfulness meditation for pain relief.* Sounds True.

Kafka, F. (1995). *The metamorphosis and other stories.* The Schocken Kafka Library. (Original work published 1915)

Kahill, S. (1988). Symptoms of professional burnout: A review of the empirical evidence. *Canadian Psychology, 29*(3), 284–297. https://doi.org/10.1037/h0079772

Kanske, P., Böckler, A., Trautwein, F.-M., & Singer, T. (2015). Dissecting the social brain: Introducing the EmpaToM to reveal distinct neural networks and brain-behavior relations for empathy and Theory of Mind. *NeuroImage, 122*, 6–19. https://doi.org/10.1016/j.neuroimage.2015.07.082

Karageorghis, C. (2008, February 12). Entering "the zone": A guide for coaches. *The Sport Journal.* https://thesportjournal.org/article/entering-the-zone-a-guide-for-coaches/

Keats, J. (2011). *The letters of John Keats to his family and friends* (S. Colvin, Ed.). Project Gutenberg. (Original work published 1891)

Kirschenbaum, H. (1979). *On becoming Carl Rogers.* Delta.

Kirschenbaum, H., & Henderson, V. L. (Eds.). (1989a). *Carl Rogers: Dialogues.* Constable.

Kirschenbaum, H., & Henderson, V. L. (Eds.). (1989b). *The Carl Rogers reader.* Houghton Mifflin.

Kleinman, A. (2019). *The soul of care.* Penguin Books.

Klimecki, O., Ricard, M., & Singer, T. (2013). Empathy versus compassion. In T. Singer & M. Bolz (Eds.), *Compassion: Bridging practice and science* (pp. 464–487). Max Planck Society. http://www.compassion-training.org/

Klimecki, O., & Singer, T. (2012). Empathic distress fatigue rather than compassion fatigue? Integrating findings from empathy research in psychology and social neuroscience. In B. Oakley, A. Knafo, G. Madhavan, & D. S. Wilson (Eds.), *Pathological altruism* (pp. 368–383). Oxford University Press.

Kohut, H. (1982). Introspection, empathy, and the semi-circle of mental health. *The International Journal of Psychoanalysis, 63*(4), 395–407.

Kongtrul, D. (2016). *The intelligent heart.* Shambhala.

Koole, S. L., & Tschacher, W. (2016, June 13). Synchrony in psychotherapy: A review and an integrative framework for the therapeutic alliance. *Frontiers in Psychology, 7*, 862. Advance online publication. https://doi.org/10.3389/fpsyg.2016.00862

Kornfield, J. (2004). *Meditation for beginners*. Sounds True.

Krol, S. A., & Bartz, J. A. (2022). The self and empathy: Lacking a clear and stable sense of self undermines empathy and helping behavior. *Emotion, 22*(7), 1554–1571. https://doi.org/10.1037/emo0000943

Kuhn, T. S. (2012). *The structure of scientific revolutions* (4th ed.). University of Chicago Press.

Kuppens, P., Tuerlinckx, F., Russell, J. A., & Barrett, L. F. (2013). The relation between valence and arousal in subjective experience. *Psychological Bulletin, 139*(4), 917–940. https://doi.org/10.1037/a0030811

Kurosawa, A. (Director). (1950). *Rashomon* [Film]. Daiei Film.

Laing, R. D. (1965). *The divided self: An existential study in sanity and madness*. Penguin Books.

Laird, J. (2000). Theorizing culture. *Journal of Feminist Family Therapy, 11*(4), 99–114. https://doi.org/10.1300/J086v11n04_08

Lakoff, G., & Johnson, M. (1980). *Metaphors we live by*. The University of Chicago Press.

Lamm, C., Decety, J., & Singer, T. (2011). Meta-analytic evidence for common and distinct neural networks associated with directly experienced pain and empathy for pain. *NeuroImage, 54*(3), 2492–2502. https://doi.org/10.1016/j.neuroimage.2010.10.014

Langer, E. J. (n.d.). *Mindfulness for everyday life*. Psychwire. https://psychwire.com/free-resources/q-and-a/1bhpwam/mindfulness-for-everyday-life

Langer, E. J. (2014). *Mindfulness*. Da Capo Press.

Langer, E. J. (2023). *The mindful body: Thinking our way to chronic health*. Ballantine Books.

Lanzoni, S. (2018). *Empathy: A history*. Yale University Press.

Lazareva, V. (2020). *When fifteen minutes is all you have: Change-focused conversation analysis of brief empathic conversations with standardized medical patients* (Publication No. 30995161) [Doctoral dissertation, Nova Southeastern University]. ProQuest Dissertations and Theses Global.

Le Guin, U. K. (2004). *The wave in the mind: Talks and essays on the writer, the reader, and the imagination*. Shambhala.

Lesté-Lasserre, C. (2019, May 2). *Horse emotions, human beliefs, and how they drive care*. The Horse. https://thehorse.com/171321/horse-emotions-human-beliefs-and-how-they-drive-care/

Lewis, K. L., & Hodges, S. D. (2012). Empathy is not always as personal as you may think: The use of stereotypes in empathic accuracy. In J. Decety (Ed.), *Empathy: From bench to bedside* (pp. 73–84). MIT Press.

Lieber, F. W. (1995). *The legacy of empathy: History of a psychological concept* (Publication No. 9601791) [Doctoral dissertation, Indiana University]. ProQuest Dissertations and Theses Global.

Lief, J. (2008). Tonglen: The practice of transformation. In S. Piver (Ed.), *Quiet mind* (pp. 65–78). Shambhala.

Lindsay, E. K., & Creswell, J. D. (2019). Mindfulness, acceptance, and emotion regulation: Perspectives from monitor and acceptance theory (MAT). *Current Opinion in Psychology, 28*, 120–125. https://doi.org/10.1016/j.copsyc.2018.12.004

Linehan, M. M. (2020). *Building a life worth living: A memoir.* Random House.

Lopez, F. G. (1987). Erickson and Rogers: The differences do make a difference. *Journal of Counseling and Development, 65*(5), 241–243. https://doi.org/10.1002/j.1556-6676.1987.tb01274.x

Lu, C. (2021, February). Dharma talks: Listening with empathy, part 3—Listen with your mind [Audio with transcript]. *Tricycle Magazine.* https://tricycle.org/dharmatalks/listening-with-empathy/

MacFarlane, P. D. (2013). *Empathy from the psychotherapy client's perspective: A qualitative examination* (Publication No. 3671561) [Doctoral dissertation, Ohio University]. ProQuest Dissertations and Theses Global.

Mahrer, A. R. (1997). Empathy as therapist–client alignment. In A. C. Bohart & L. S. Greenberg (Eds.), *Empathy reconsidered: New directions in psychotherapy* (pp. 187–213). American Psychological Association. https://doi.org/10.1037/10226-008

Maibom, H. L. (Ed.). (2017). *The Routledge handbook of philosophy of empathy.* Taylor & Francis. https://doi.org/10.4324/9781315282015

Maibom, H. L. (2022). *The space between: How empathy really works.* Oxford University Press. https://doi.org/10.1093/oso/9780197637081.001.0001

Makransky, J. (2012). Compassion in Buddhist psychology. In R. D. Siegel & C. K. Germer (Eds.), *Wisdom and compassion in psychotherapy* (pp. 61–78). Guilford Press.

Margulies, A. (1989). *The empathic imagination.* Norton.

Maxwell, I., Seton, M., & Szabó, M. (2015). The Australian actors' wellbeing study: A preliminary report. *About Performance, 13*, 69–113. https://search.informit.org/doi/10.3316/informit.499926749273237

McCall, C., Steinbeis, N., Ricard, M., & Singer, T. (2014, December 8). Compassion meditators show less anger, less punishment, and more compensation of victims in response to fairness violations. *Frontiers in Behavioral Neuroscience, 8*, 424. https://doi.org/10.3389/fnbeh.2014.00424

McCann, I. L., & Pearlman, L. A. (1990). Vicarious traumatization: A framework for understanding the psychological effects of working with victims. *Journal of Traumatic Stress, 3*(1), 131–149. https://doi.org/10.1007/BF00975140

McClintock, A. S., Anderson, T., Patterson, C. L., & Wing, E. H. (2018). Early psychotherapeutic empathy, alliance, and client outcome: Preliminary evidence of indirect effects. *Journal of Clinical Psychology, 74*(6), 839–848. https://doi.org/10.1002/jclp.22568

McIntyre, S. L., Samstag, L. W., Haden, S. C., & Duncan, J. W. (2019). Therapist experience, personal therapy, and distressing states of mind: Regulation and resonance as dialectics of therapeutic empathy. *Journal of Contemporary Psychotherapy, 49*(4), 213–221. https://doi.org/10.1007/s10879-019-09431-w

McLaren, K. (2013). *The art of empathy*. Sounds True.

Meador, B. D., & Rogers, C. R. (1984). Person-centered therapy. In R. Corsini (Ed.), *Current psychotherapies* (3rd ed., pp. 142–195). F. E. Peacock.

Meares, R. (1983, February). Keats and the "impersonal" therapist: A note on empathy and the therapeutic screen. *Psychiatry, 46*(1), 73–82. https://doi.org/10.1080/00332747.1983.11024179

Meissner, W. W. (2010). Some notes on the epistemology of empathy. *The Psychoanalytic Quarterly, 79*(2), 421–469. https://doi.org/10.1002/j.2167-4086.2010.tb00454.x

Mesquita, B. (2022). *Between us: How cultures create emotions*. Norton.

Miller, J. A. (1989, March). Wonder as hinge. *International Philosophical Quarterly, 29*(1), 53–66. https://doi.org/10.5840/ipq198929146

Miller, S. D., Hubble, M. A., & Chow, D. (2020). *Better results: Using deliberate practice to improve therapeutic effectiveness*. American Psychological Association. https://doi.org/10.1037/0000191-000

Mina, D. (2023, August 26). Stepping into Raymond Chandler's shoes showed me the power of fiction. *The New York Times*. https://www.nytimes.com/2023/08/26/opinion/raymond-chandler-philip-marlowe-denise-mina.html

Mirzaei Maghsud, A., Abazari, F., Miri, S., & Sadat Nematollahi, M. (2020). The effectiveness of empathy training on the empathy skills of nurses working in intensive care units. *Journal of Research in Nursing, 25*(8), 722–731. https://doi.org/10.1177/1744987120902827

Mumford, G. (2015). *The mindful athlete: Secrets to pure performance*. Parallax Press.

Nachmanovitch, S. (2019). *The art of is: Improvising as a way of life*. New World Library.

Nagel, T. (1974, October). What is it like to be a bat? *The Philosophical Review, 83*(4), 435–450. https://doi.org/10.2307/2183914

NBC. (2022, February 27). *When Beth falls, she gets back up | NBC's This Is Us*. https://www.nbc.com/this-is-us/video/when-beth-falls-she-gets-back-up-nbcs-this-is-us/HaZ75KTul0V1lY1Ue5X_OfD6blZPSb_0

Neff, K. D. (2012). The science of self-compassion. In R. D. Siegel & C. K. Germer (Eds.), *Wisdom and compassion in psychotherapy* (pp. 79–92). Guilford Press.

Neukrug, E. (2017, February). *Creative and novel approaches to empathy*. Counseling Today Archive. https://ctarchive.counseling.org/2017/02/creative-novel-approaches-empathy/

Nguyen, B. (Director). (2024). *The greatest night in pop* [Film]. Republic Pictures; Dorothy Street Pictures; MRC; MakeMake Entertainment.

Nienhuis, J. B., Owen, J., Valentine, J. C., Winkeljohn Black, S., Halford, T. C., Parazak, S. E., Budge, S., & Hilsenroth, M. (2018). Therapeutic alliance, empathy, and genuineness in individual adult psychotherapy: A meta-analytic review. *Psychotherapy Research, 28*(4), 593–605. https://doi.org/10.1080/10503307.2016.1204023

Norcross, J. C., & Lambert, M. J. (2018). Psychotherapy relationships that work III. *Psychotherapy, 55*(4), 303–315. https://doi.org/10.1037/pst0000193

Norton, M. (2024). *The ritual effect.* Scribner.

Nussbaum, M. C. (2001). *Upheavals of thought: The intelligence of emotions.* Cambridge University Press. https://doi.org/10.1017/CBO9780511840715

O'Hanlon, B., & Bertolino, B. (1998). *Invitation to possibility land: An intensive teaching seminar with Bill O'Hanlon.* Routledge.

O'Hara, M. (1997). Relational empathy: Beyond modernist egocentricism to postmodern holistic contextualism. In A. C. Bohart & L. S. Greenberg (Eds.), *Empathy reconsidered: New directions in psychotherapy* (pp. 295–319). American Psychological Association. https://doi.org/10.1037/10226-013

Olendzki, A. (2005). The roots of mindfulness. In C. K. Germer, R. D. Siegel, & P. R. Fulton (Eds.), *Mindfulness and psychotherapy* (pp. 241–261). Guilford Press.

Olendzki, A. (2010). *Unlimiting mind.* Wisdom Publications.

Oliver, L. D. (2017). *Function and dysfunction in distinct facets of empathy* (Publication No. 2714865637) [Doctoral dissertation, University of Western Ontario]. ProQuest Dissertations and Theses Global.

Osler, W. (1904). *Aequanimitas and other addresses.* H. K. Lewis. https://archive.org/details/b24757767

Palubeckas, A. J. (1981). *Rapport in the therapeutic relationship and its relationship to pacing* (Publication No. 303203156) [Doctoral dissertation, Boston University]. ProQuest Dissertations and Theses Global.

Paz, L. V., Viola, T. W., Milanesi, B. B., Sulzbach, J. H., Mestriner, R. G., Wieck, A., & Xavier, L. L. (2022, March). Contagious depression: Automatic mimicry and the mirror neuron system—A review. *Neuroscience and Biobehavioral Reviews, 134,* Article 104509. https://doi.org/10.1016/j.neubiorev.2021.12.032

Pearlman, L. A., & Saakvitne, K. W. (1995). Treating therapists with vicarious traumatization and secondary traumatic stress disorder. In C. R. Figley (Ed.), *Compassion fatigue: Coping with secondary traumatic stress disorder in those who treat the traumatized* (pp. 150–177). Routledge.

Pedersen, P. B., Crethar, H. C., & Carlson, J. (2008). *Inclusive cultural empathy: Making relationships central in counseling and psychotherapy.* American Psychological Association. https://doi.org/10.1037/11707-000

Pence, G. E. (1983). Can compassion be taught? *Journal of Medical Ethics, 9*(4), 189–191. https://doi.org/10.1136/jme.9.4.189

Perry, R. (1993). Empathy—Still at the heart of therapy: The interplay of context and therapy. *Australian and New Zealand Journal of Family Therapy, 14*(2), 63–74. https://doi.org/10.1002/j.1467-8438.1993.tb00943.x

Phelps, C. (2024, June 8). Caitlin Clark's unique free throw ritual captivates fans. *Athlon Sports.* https://athlonsports.com/wnba/caitlin-clark-free-throw-ritual-captivates-wnba-fans

Phelps-Thiry, C. (1996). *The relationship of family and individual perceived therapist empathy to outcome in brief family therapy* (Publication No. 9713887) [Doctoral dissertation, Columbia University]. ProQuest Dissertations and Theses Global.

Pigman, G. W. (1995). Freud and the history of empathy. *The International Journal of Psychoanalysis, 76*(2), 237–256.

Pollak, K. I., & Ashton-James, C. (2018). Empathy is not empathy is not empathy in the management of chronic pain. *Patient Education and Counseling, 101*(12), 2045–2046. https://doi.org/10.1016/j.pec.2018.10.008

Popova, M. (2015, January 20). *Mary Oliver on what attention really means and her moving elegy for her soul mate*. The Marginalian. https://www.themarginalian.org/2015/01/20/mary-oliver-molly-malone-cook-our-world/

Preckel, K., Kanske, P., & Singer, T. (2018, February). On the interaction of social affect and cognition: Empathy, compassion and theory of mind. *Current Opinion in Behavioral Sciences, 19*, 1–6. https://doi.org/10.1016/j.cobeha.2017.07.010

Preston, S. D., Bechara, A., Damasio, H., Grabowski, T. J., Stansfield, R. B., Mehta, S., & Damasio, A. R. (2007). The neural substrates of cognitive empathy. *Social Neuroscience, 2*(3–4), 254–275. https://doi.org/10.1080/17470910701376902

Preston, S. D., & de Waal, F. B. M. (2002). Empathy: Its ultimate and proximate bases. *Behavioral and Brain Sciences, 25*(1), 1–20. https://doi.org/10.1017/S0140525X02000018

Prinz, J. (2011). Against empathy [Special issue]. *The Southern Journal of Philosophy, 49*(s1), 214–233. https://doi.org/10.1111/j.2041-6962.2011.00069.x

Raingruber, B. J. (2001). Settling into and moving in a climate of care: Styles and patterns of interaction between nurse psychotherapists and clients. *Perspectives in Psychiatric Care, 37*(1), 15–27. https://doi.org/10.1111/j.1744-6163.2001.tb00612.x

Rautalinko, E., & Lisper, H.-O. (2004). Effects of training reflective listening in a corporate setting. *Journal of Business and Psychology, 18*(3), 281–299. https://doi.org/10.1023/B:JOBU.0000016712.36043.4f

Rautalinko, E., Lisper, H.-O., & Ekehammar, B. (2007). Reflective listening in counseling: Effects of training time and evaluator social skills. *American Journal of Psychotherapy, 61*(2), 191–209. https://doi.org/10.1176/appi.psychotherapy.2007.61.2.191

Reik, T. (1948). *Listening with the third ear*. Arena Books.

Remnick, D. (Host). (2017, November 24). Bruce Springsteen talks with David Remnick [Audio podcast episode]. In *The New Yorker Radio Hour*. https://www.newyorker.com/podcast/the-new-yorker-radio-hour/bruce-springsteen-talks-with-david-remnick

Ricard, M. (2010). *Why meditate?* Hay House.

Ricard, M., & Singer, W. (2017). *Beyond the self: Conversations between Buddhism and Neuroscience*. MIT Press. https://doi.org/10.7551/mitpress/11376.001.0001

Rieber, R. W. (Ed.). (1989). *The individual, communication, and society: Essays in memory of Gregory Bateson*. Cambridge University Press.

Rogers, C. R. (1942). The use of electrically recorded interviews in improving psychotherapeutic techniques. *American Journal of Orthopsychiatry, 12*(3), 429–434. https://doi.org/10.1111/j.1939-0025.1942.tb05930.x

Rogers, C. R. (1952). A personal formulation of client-centered therapy. *Marriage and Family Living, 14*(4), 341–361. https://doi.org/10.2307/348729

Rogers, C. R. (1957). The necessary and sufficient conditions of therapeutic personality change. *Journal of Consulting Psychology, 21*(2), 95–103. https://doi.org/10.1037/h0045357

Rogers, C. R. (1959). A theory of therapy, personality, and interpersonal relationships, as developed in the client-centered framework. In S. Koch (Ed.), *Psychology: A study of a science: Study 1, Vol. 3. Formulations of the person and the social context* (pp. 184–256). McGraw Hill.

Rogers, C. R. (1962). The interpersonal relationship: The core of guidance. *Harvard Educational Review, 32*(4), 416–429.

Rogers, C. R. (1975). Empathic: An unappreciated way of being. *The Counseling Psychologist, 5*(2), 2–10. https://doi.org/10.1177/001100007500500202

Rogers, C. R. (1980). *A way of being*. Houghton Mifflin.

Rogers, C. R. (1987). Rogers, Kohut, and Erickson: A personal perspective on some similarities and differences. In J. K. Zeig (Ed.), *The evolution of psychotherapy* (pp. 179 187). Brunner/Mazel.

Rogers, C. R. (1989a). The necessary and sufficient conditions of therapeutic personality change. In H. Kirschenbaum & V. L. Henderson (Eds.), *The Carl Rogers reader* (pp. 219–235). Houghton Mifflin. https://doi.org/10.1080/1046171X.1989.12034347

Rogers, C. R. (1989b). Reflection of feelings and transference. In H. Kirschenbaum & V. L. Henderson (Eds.), *The Carl Rogers reader* (pp. 127–134). Houghton Mifflin.

Rogers, C. R. (2007). The basic conditions of the facilitative therapeutic relationship. In M. Cooper, M. O'Hara, P. F. Schmid, & G. Wyatt (Eds.), *The handbook of person-centered psychotherapy and counselling* (pp. 1–5). Palgrave Macmillan.

Rogers, C. R., & Farson, R. E. (2021). *Active listening*. Mockingbird Press. (Original work published 1957)

Rogers, C. R., & Roethlisberger, F. J. (1952, July/August). Barriers and gateways to communication. *Harvard Business Review*, 46–52.

Rosengren, D. B. (2009). *Building motivational interviewing skills: A practitioner workbook*. Guilford Press.

Rowling, J. K. (1998). *Harry Potter and the sorcerer's stone*. Scholastic Press.

Rumi. (1994). The guest house (C. Barks, Trans.). In *Rumi: Selected poems* (p. 109). Penguin Books. (Original work published ca. 1250)

Ruthven, K. K. (1969). The poet as etymologist. *Critical Quarterly, 11*(1), 9–37. https://doi.org/10.1111/j.1467-8705.1969.tb02229.x

Sacks, H., Schegloff, E., & Jefferson, G. (1974). A simple systematic for the organisation of turn taking in conversation. *Language, 50*(4), 696–735. https://doi.org/10.1353/lan.1974.0010

Salzberg, S. (2011). *Real happiness: The power of meditation.* Workman Publishing.

Saunders, G. (2021). *A swim in a pond in the rain.* Random House.

Schaefer, J. (Host). (2007, September 19). Leo Kottke [Audio podcast episode]. In *Sound check with John Schaefer.* https://www.newsounds.org/story/39959-leo-kottke/

Schulman, M. (2021, December 5). On "Succession," Jeremy Strong doesn't get the joke. *The New Yorker.* https://www.newyorker.com/magazine/2021/12/13/on-succession-jeremy-strong-doesnt-get-the-joke

Seabrook, J. (2023, June 5). The case for and against Ed Sheeran. *The New Yorker.* https://www.newyorker.com/magazine/2023/06/05/ed-sheeran-copyright-infringement-lawsuit-marvin-gaye

Segal, E. A., Gerdes, K. E., Lietz, C. A., Wagaman, M. A., & Geiger, J. M. (2017). *Assessing empathy.* Columbia University Press.

Seikkula, J., Karvonen, A., Kykyri, V. L., Penttonen, M., & Nyman-Salonen, P. (2018). The relational mind in couple therapy: A Bateson-inspired view of human life as an embodied stream. *Family Process, 57*(4), 855–866. https://doi.org/10.1111/famp.12382

Selvini Palazzoli, M., Boscolo, L., Cecchin, G., & Prata, G. (1978). *Paradox and counterparadox* (E. V. Burt, Trans.). Jason Aronson. (Original work published 1975)

Selvini Palazzoli, M., Boscolo, L., Cecchin, G., & Prata, G. (1980). Hypothesizing—Circularity—Neutrality: Three guidelines for the conductor of the session. *Family Process, 19*(1), 3–12. https://doi.org/10.1111/j.1545-5300.1980.00003.x

Seton, M. C. (2008). "Post-dramatic stress": Negotiating vulnerability for performance. In I. Maxwell (Ed.), *Being there: After—Proceedings of the 2006 conference of the Australasian Association for Drama, Theatre and Performance Studies.* University of Sydney. http://ses.library.usyd.edu.au/handle/2123/2518

Shaheen, J. (Host). (2023, September 13). Don't despair of this falling world: Interview with Jane Hirshfield (No. 92) [Audio podcast episode]. In *Tricycle Talks.* https://open.spotify.com/episode/2Gx2oS0OnexIxsennzSKe4?go=1&sp_cid=74418b4d5d715c42c8c93bbfc335aaff&utm_source=embed_player_p&utm_medium=desktop&nd=1&dlsi=60002a827d3340fb

Shakespeare, W. (2011). *The complete works.* Latus ePublishing. (Original work published 1599)

Shamay-Tsoory, S. G. (2009). Empathic processing: Its cognitive and affective dimensions and neuroanatomical basis. In J. Decety & W. Ickes (Eds.), *The social neuroscience of empathy* (pp. 215–232). MIT Press. https://doi.org/10.7551/mitpress/9780262012973.003.0017

Shapiro, J. (2012). The paradox of teaching empathy in medical education. In J. Decety (Ed.), *Empathy: From bench to bedside* (pp. 275–290). MIT Press.

Sharf, Z. (2024, December 23). Adrien Brody has PTSD from 'The Pianist' weight loss; his near-starvation diet made him 129 pounds for filming: 'That was necessary for storytelling'. *Variety.* https://variety.com/2024/film/news/adrien-brody-ptsd-pianist-weight-loss-starvation-diet-1236257762/

Shlien, J. (1961). A client-centered approach to schizophrenia: First approximation. In A. Burton (Ed.), *Psychotherapy of the psychoses* (pp. 285–317). Basic Books. https://doi.org/10.1037/10643-010

Shlien, J. (1997). Empathy in psychotherapy: A vital mechanism? Yes. Therapist's conceit? All too often. By itself enough? No. In A. C. Bohart & L. S. Greenberg (Eds.), *Empathy reconsidered: New directions in psychotherapy* (pp. 63–80). American Psychological Association. https://doi.org/10.1037/10226-002

Shotter, J. (2005). Goethe and the refiguring of intellectual inquiry: From 'aboutness'-thinking to 'withness'-thinking in everyday life. *Janus Head, 8*(1), 132–158. https://doi.org/10.5840/jh20058141

Siegel, D. J. (2010). *Mindsight: The new science of personal transformation.* Bantam Books.

Siegel, R. D., & Germer, C. K. (2012). Wisdom and compassion: Two wings of a bird. In R. D. Siegel & C. K. Germer (Eds.), *Wisdom and compassion in psychotherapy* (pp. 7–34). Guilford Press.

Singer, T., & Bolz, M. (Eds.). (2013). *Compassion: Bridging practice and science.* Max Planck Society. http://www.compassion-training.org/

Singer, T., & Lamm, C. (2009). The social neuroscience of empathy. *Annals of the New York Academy of Sciences, 1156*(1), 81–96. https://doi.org/10.1111/j.1749-6632.2009.04418.x

Smith, A. (1759). *The theory of moral sentiments.*

Smith, A. (2006). Cognitive empathy and emotional empathy in human behavior and evolution. *The Psychological Record, 56*(1), 3–21. https://doi.org/10.1007/BF03395534

Smith, M. (2011). Empathy, expansionism, and the extended mind. In A. Coplan & P. Goldie (Eds.), *Empathy: Philosophical and psychological perspectives* (pp. 99–117). Oxford University Press. https://doi.org/10.1093/acprof:oso/9780199539956.003.0008

Soloski, A. (2023, December 1). Elizabeth Debicki hasn't let go of Princess Diana. *The New York Times.* https://www.nytimes.com/2023/12/01/arts/television/the-crown-elizabeth-debicki-diana.html

Soto-Rubio, A., & Sinclair, S. (2018, May). In defense of sympathy, in consideration of empathy, and in praise of compassion: A history of the present. *Journal of Pain and Symptom Management, 55*(5), 1428–1434. https://doi.org/10.1016/j.jpainsymman.2017.12.478

Spaulding, S. (2017). Cognitive empathy. In H. L. Maibom (Ed.), *The Routledge handbook of philosophy of empathy* (pp. 13–21). Taylor & Francis. https://doi.org/10.4324/9781315282015-2

Storer, C. (Writer), Calo, J. (Writer), & Storer, C. (Director). (2022, June 23). Braciole (Season 1, Episode 8) [TV series episode]. In J. Calo, N. Matteson, H. Murai, J. Senior, & C. Storer (Executive Producers), *The Bear*. FX.

Stotland, E. (1969). Exploratory investigations of empathy. *Advances in Experimental Social Psychology, 4*, 271–314. https://doi.org/10.1016/S0065-2601(08)60080-5

Stueber, K. R. (2006). *Rediscovering empathy: Agency, folk psychology, and the human sciences*. MIT Press. https://doi.org/10.7551/mitpress/5833.001.0001

Sudnow, D. (1978). *Ways of the hand*. Bantam Books.

Sundararajan, L. (1995). Echoes after Carl Rogers: "Reflective listening" revisited. *The Humanistic Psychologist, 23*(2), 259–271. https://doi.org/10.1080/08873267.1995.9986828

Sutherland, O. (2005). A family therapist's constructionist perspective on the therapeutic relationship. *Journal of Systemic Therapies, 24*(2), 1–17. https://doi.org/10.1521/jsyt.2005.24.2.1

Suzuki, S. (2006). *Zen mind, beginner's mind*. Shambhala.

Ta, V. P., & Ickes, W. (2017). Empathic accuracy. In H. L. Maibom (Ed.), *The Routledge handbook of philosophy of empathy* (pp. 353–363). Taylor & Francis. https://doi.org/10.4324/9781315282015-32

Taylor, L. (2017, December 6). Out of character: How acting puts a mental strain on performers. *The Conversation*. https://theconversation.com/out-of-character-how-acting-puts-a-mental-strain-on-performers-86212

Thomas, L. (1990). *Etcetera, etcetera: Notes of a word-watcher*. Penguin.

Timmers, I., Park, A. L., Fischer, M. D., Kronman, C. A., Heathcote, L. C., Hernandez, J. M., & Simons, L. E. (2018, November 26). Is empathy for pain unique in its neural correlates? A meta-analysis of neuroimaging studies of empathy. *Frontiers in Behavioral Neuroscience, 12*, 289. Advance online publication. https://doi.org/10.3389/fnbeh.2018.00289

Travers, P. L. (2014). *Mary Poppins: 80th anniversary collection*. Houghton Mifflin Harcourt. (Original work published 1934)

Truax, C. B., & Carkhuff, R. R. (1967). *Toward effective counseling and psychotherapy*. Aldine.

Truax, C. B., & Lister, J. L. (1970). The effects of counselor accurate empathy and non-possessive warmth upon client vocational rehabilitation progress. *Conseiller Canadien, 4*(4), 229–232.

Uhrig, A. (2018). *Exploring empathy in medical narratives* [Master's thesis, Northern Michigan University]. MNU Commons. https://commons.nmu.edu/theses/560

United Nations. (n.d.). *Discussion phase: General debate*. https://www.un.org/en/model-united-nations/discussion-phase-general-debate

van Baaren, R. B., Decety, J., Dijksterhuis, A., van de Leij, A., & van Leeuwen, M. L. (2009). Being imitated: Consequences of nonconsciously showing empathy. In J. Decety & W. Ickes (Eds.), *The social neuroscience of empathy* (pp. 31–42). MIT Press. https://doi.org/10.7551/mitpress/9780262012973.003.0004

Wampold, B. E., & Imel, Z. E. (2015). *The great psychotherapy debate: Evidence for what makes psychotherapy work* (2nd ed.). Routledge. https://doi.org/10.4324/9780203582015

Warren, J. (n.d.). *Welcome to the party* [Audio meditation]. Happier.

Waters, M. (Director). (2003). *Freaky Friday* [Film]. Walt Disney Pictures; Gunn Films.

Watson, J. C., & Greenberg, L. S. (2011). Empathic resonance: A neuroscience perspective. In J. Decety & W. Ickes (Eds.), *The social neuroscience of empathy* (pp. 125–137). MIT Press.

Watson, J. C., Steckley, P. L., & McMullen, E. J. (2014). The role of empathy in promoting change. *Psychotherapy Research*, *24*(3), 286–298. https://doi.org/10.1080/10503307.2013.802823

Watson, S. K. (Writer), Freeman, E. (Writer), & Hook, K. (Director). (2022, February 22). Our little island girl: Part two (Season 6, Episode 6) [TV series episode]. In D. Fogelman, J. Rosenthal, E. Berger, G. Ficarra, C. Gogolak, J. Requa, I. Aptaker, & K. Olin (Executive Producers), *This is us*. Rhode Island Ave. Productions, Zaftig Films, and 20th Television.

Watts, A. (1975). *Tao: The watercourse way*. Pantheon books.

Watzlawick, P., Weakland, J., & Fisch, R. (1974). *Change: Principles of problem formation and problem resolution*. Norton.

We Are the World. (2024, December). In *Wikipedia*. https://en.wikipedia.org/w/index.php?title=We_Are_the_World&oldid=1265462780

Whitaker, C. A., & Bumberry, W. M. (1988). *Dancing with the family: A symbolic experiential approach*. Bruner Mazel.

Wilkinson, M. (1992). How do we understand empathy systemically? *Journal of Family Therapy*, *14*(2), 193–205. https://doi.org/10.1046/j..1992.00452.x

Willroth, E. C., Young, G., Tamir, M., & Mauss, I. B. (2023). Judging emotions as good or bad: Individual differences and associations with psychological health. *Emotion*, *23*(7), 1876–1890. https://doi.org/10.1037/emo0001220

Winkler, H., & Rich, J. (Executive Producers). (1985–1992). *MacGyver* [TV series]. Henry Winkler–John Rich Productions; Paramount Network Television.

Wispé, L. (1986). The distinction between sympathy and empathy: To call forth a concept, a word is needed. *Journal of Personality and Social Psychology*, *50*(2), 314–321. https://doi.org/10.1037/0022-3514.50.2.314

Wispé, L. (1987). History of the concept of empathy. In N. Eisenberg & J. Strayer (Eds.), *Empathy and its development* (pp. 17–37). Cambridge University Press.

Wittgenstein, L. (1953). *Philosophical investigations* (E. Anscombe, Trans.). Macmillan.

Wittgenstein, L. (1980). *Culture and value* (G. H. von Wright & H. Nyman, Eds.; P. Winch, Trans.). The University of Chicago Press.

Woolf, V. (1931). *The waves*. Harcourt.

Yalom, I. (2002). *The gift of therapy*. HarperCollins.

Zahavi, D., & Overgaard, S. (2012). Empathy without isomorphism: A phenomenological account. In J. Decety (Ed.), *Empathy: From bench to bedside* (pp. 3–20). MIT Press.

Zaki, J. (2014). Empathy: A motivated account. *Psychological Bulletin, 140*(6), 1608–1647. https://doi.org/10.1037/a0037679

Zaki, J. (2019). *The war for kindness: Building empathy in a fractured world*. Broadway Books.

Zaki, J., Bolger, N., & Ochsner, K. (2008). It takes two: The interpersonal nature of empathic accuracy. *Psychological Science, 19*(4), 399–404. https://doi.org/10.1111/j.1467-9280.2008.02099.x

Zaki, J., & Ochsner, K. (2011). Reintegrating the study of accuracy into social cognition research. *Psychological Inquiry, 22*(3), 159–182. https://doi.org/10.1080/1047840X.2011.551743

Zaki, J., Wager, T. D., Singer, T., Keysers, C., & Gazzola, V. (2016). The anatomy of suffering: Understanding the relationship between nociceptive and empathic pain. *Trends in Cognitive Sciences, 20*(4), 249–259. https://doi.org/10.1016/j.tics.2016.02.003

Zaretsky, R. (2021). *The subversive Simone Weil: A life in five ideas*. The University of Chicago Press.

Index

A

Accurate empathy, 52, 145
Accurate reflection, 130
Activation, 50
Active listening, 4, 100, 145
Actors, 88–90
"Aesthetic projection," as original conception of Einfühlung, 24
Affect, 48–49
Affective empathy, 44–46, 48–49, 53
Allostasis, 50
Analogy-inflected empathy, 57
Anderson, R., 65
Andreescu, Bianca, 77
Anthropomorphism, 58
Aragno, A., 11, 119
Aristotle, 48
Arousal, 50
As–if clause, Rogers's, 70
Asking questions, 140–145
Asymmetry
　of complementarity, 98
　of empathic conversations, 67
　of empathic relationships, 69
　of metaphor, 67
　of therapeutic relationships, 69
Attitude, and technique, 127
Attunement, 122

B

Baldwin, James Mark, 26
Barrett, L. F., 11, 41, 48–54, 86, 103
Basic emotions, 49
Bateson, G., 48, 59, 66–67, 75, 94, 120, 123–124, 147n3

Bateson, M. C., 59
Batson, C. D., 18, 25, 29, 75
The Bear (TV series), 146
Beginner's mind, 104–105
Belafonte, Harry, 63
Benefits of redundancy, 120–125
Bergen, Benjamin K., 60
Besman-Albinder, S., 74
Bias, 43
Blake, W., 51
Bloom, P., 20, 26–27, 29, 48
Bochner, A., vii
Body-based self identity, 13
Bohart, A. C., 131, 140
Borke, H., 46
Both–and empathizing, 151–157
Boundaries, self–other, 56
Bozarth, J. D., 52
Bridges, J., 64–65
Brody, Adrien, 88
Brown, B., 114
Bryant, Kobe, 77
Buber, M., 19, 65, 69–70
Buddhism, 34, 36–37. *See also* Tonglen
Burnout, 35–37

C

Carmen Berzatto (fictional character), 146
Carroll, L., 19
Carson, Johnny, 56
Charles, Ray, 63
Certainty, 54, 94, 100, 103, 104, 105, 117
Chödrön, P., 37, 69, 73

189

Circumscribed self, 16, 62, 63, 65, 112, 114
Circumscribed sense of self, 31, 57, 76
Cissna, K. N., 65
Claiming, 114–117
Clark, Caitlin, 91
Classical model of emotion, 49–50
Cognition, 48–49
Cognitive empathy, 44, 46–49, 53
Cohen, T., vii, 61
Collecting, and releasing, 81–82
Compassion, 33–40
   empathy and sympathy vs., 17–21
   fatigue, 35–37, 74
   as term, 33
Complementarity, of relationships, 66–67
Concern
   detached, 36
   sympathetic, 29–31
Conscious, as term, 121
Constructed emotion theory, 49–52
   vs. classical model, 49, 50, 51, 130
Contagion, emotional, 19, 25, 26, 27, 31, 45
Coplan, A., 24, 31, 49, 58, 60
Cordaro, D., 49
Counseling and Psychotherapy (Rogers), 130
Cox, Brian, 89
Creswell, J. D., 83
Crichton, M., 75
Crouch, Andy, 121
The Crown (TV series), 89
Csikszentmihalyi, M., 63
Curiosity. *See* Empathic curiosity
Curry, Stephen, 77
Curtis, Jamie Lee, 62n5

D

Dark empathy, 40
Day-Lewis, Daniel, 88–89
Debicki, Elizabeth, 89
Decety, J., 74–75
Decristofaro, Jason, 127
Dehumanization, 74
Delgado, N., 35
Depth of meaning, 125
De-roling, 88–92
de Saussure, F., 20
Descartes, R., 48
Detached concern, 36
De Waal, F. B. M., 24–25

Diana, Princess of Wales, 89
Distress, personal, 31–33
Double description, 123–124
Dovetail complementarity, 70, 95, 98
Dovetail metaphor, for empathy, 67, 95
Duncan, S., 48
Dunning, D., 100
Durrell, L., 152
Dylan, Bob, 63
Dymond, R. F., 46

E

Einfühlung, 21–23, 60
Ekman, P., 49
Elliott, R., 56, 139
Ellis, Carolyn, xi, 6, 11, 12, 18, 25, 29, 31, 35, 45
Emotional empathy, 44
Emotions, 27, 48–52
Empath, 28, 90
   vs. "sympath," 28, 90n5
Empathic accuracy, 52–55, 130. *See also* Accurate empathy
Empathic concern, 25
Empathic curiosity, 41–71
   affective empathy, 45–46
   cognition and affect, 48–49
   cognitive empathy, 46–48
   empathic accuracy, 52–55
   in-the-shoes imagination, 56–59
   metaphoric imagination, 59–62
   relational shape of empathy, 66–71
   self-less imagination, 63–66
   sparking the empathic imagination, 55–56
   theory of constructed emotion, 49–52
Empathic depth conception, 125
Empathic disengagement, 163
Empathic imagination, 55–56
Empathic knowing, 44
Empathic listening, 128–137
Empathy, 23–25. *See also* Skills of empathic engagement
   affect-attenuated (i.e., cognitive), 49, 53, 55
   affective, 44–46, 48–49, 53
   analogy-inflected, 57, 96n1
   both–and, 151–157
   cognition-attenuated (i.e., affective), 49, 53
   cognitive, 44, 46–49, 53
   compassion and sympathy vs., 17–21

dark, 40
dovetail metaphor for, 67, 95
emotional, 44
relational shape of, 66–71
selective, 113
as term, 19–24
Empathy-inflected sympathy, 30
Engagement, 77–81
Epstein, Mark, 63
Epstein, R., 46, 51, 92, 96
Equanimity,36
Equanimity, Buddhist, 36, 37, 38
Equanimity, Osler-style, 36, 38
Erickson, M. H., 91, 112–113, 148–149
Erickson, Robert, 148–149
Error correction, 137–140, 160
Eyal, T., 54

F

Facial movements, 51, 53
"Feel for," 30, 31, 32, 37, 39
"Feel with" (etymology of sympathy), 25, 26, 29, 31, 33, 35, 152
Feeling, 44
"Feeling one's way into," 3, 21, 22, 75, 88
Fiennes, Ralph, 111–112
Firestein, S., 100, 105, 137
Fischer, N., 16, 38, 39, 66
Fish, Stanley, 43
Fitzgerald, F. S., 151, 152
Fitzgerald, Faith T., 43
Flaskas, C., 60, 102
Floating hunches, 140–145
Flow, 63
Folsom, Ed, 41n1
Fox, Renée, 36
Friedman, M., 65
Fuller, Buckminster, 147
Functional MRI (fMRI), 38

G

Gaye, Marvin, 106
Geller, S. M., 45
Gendlin, E. T., 125, 145
German philosophy, 21–23
Germer, C. K., 38
Glassman, B., 64–65, 128
Gleichgerrcht, E., 74–75
Goeth, Amon, 111
Goldie, P., 26

Goldman, Alvin I. (2011), 47
Gordon, M., 79
The Greatest Night in Pop (documentary), 64
Green, Shelley, 97, 107, 122
Greenberg, L. S., 56
Greenleaf, Eric, 90
"The Grey Monk" (Blake), 51

H

Halpern, J., 43, 56, 58, 129, 139, 141
Handwashing, 90–91
Harrington, A., 33
Herder, Johann Gottfried von, 21–22
Hippocrates, 48
Hirschfield, J., 63, 73, 105
Hodges, S. D., 54
Houshmand, Z., 37
Humpty Dumpty, 19–20
Hunches, 140

I

Ickes, W., 52, 54
Ignorance, 99–102
Imagination
  in-the-shoes, 56–59
  self-less, 63–66
Imagination-enhanced mindfulness meditation, 86–88
"Imagine–other" scenario, 32
"Imagine–self" scenario, 31–32
Imperturbability, 36
Including, and learning, 84–86
Interlacing, 145–151
Interoception, 50
Interpersonal error correction, 160
In-the-shoes imagination, 56–59
I–thou relationship, empathy as, 69

J

Jackson, Michael, 63
James, Lebron, 77
Jamison, L., 23, 49, 103, 125, 140
Jinpa, T., 34
Joel, Billy, 63
The Jolson Story (film), 89
Jones, Quincy, 63–64, 66
Jordan, Michael, 77
Judging, 107–114

K

Kabat-Zinn, J., 75, 77
Kanske, P., 37
Kastor, Deena, 77
Kaufmann, Walter, 23
Keats, J., 63
Kendall Roy (fictional character), 89
Kleinman, A., 74
Klimecki, O., 30, 37
Know, as term, 44
Kohut, H., 39
Kottke, Leo, 63
Kurosawa, A., 152

L

Laing, R. D., 12
Langer, E. J., 56, 107, 124, 135
Lanzoni, S., vii, 60, 65
Lao Tzu, 99
The Last of the Mohicans (film), 88
Lauper, Cyndi, 63
Learning, 84–86
Leave-taking, 163
Lee, Vernon (Violet Paget), 22
Le Guin, U. K., 55, 128
Lewis, Huey, 63
Lewis, K. L., 54
Lieber, F. W., 17
Lief, J., 74
Lindsay, E. K., 83
Lipps, T., 22, 60, 62
Listening, 130–137
Lloyd, Carli, 77
Logan Roy (fictional character), 89
Loggins, Kenny, 63
Lohan, Lindsay, 62n5
Lord Voldemort (fictional character), 111

M

Mahrer, A. R., 60
Maibom, H. L., 28, 43, 54, 57, 61, 121
Makransky, J., 34
Margulies, A., 141
Mary Poppins (fictional character), 159
May, Rollo, 62, 127
McIntyre, S. L., 75
McLaren, K., 28
Meador, B. D., 137
Meaning, depth of, 125

Meditation, 77–79
  mindfulness meditation, 28, 66, 77, 78, 79, 80, 81, 83, 86, 90, 107, 114
  narration of mindfulness meditation, 15
Meissner, W. W., 61
Mesquita, B., 51
Meta-ignorance, 100–101
Metaphor, concept of, 59, 60, 61, 62, 67
Metaphorical identity, 67
Metaphoric imagination, 59–62
Milan Systemic Therapy team, 154
Miller, J. A., 93, 103
Mindful disengagement, 88–92
Mindful engagement. *See* Therapist self-care
Mindfulness, 76–83, 86–88
Mindfulness-Based Stress Reduction Clinic, 77
Multipartiality, 43, 154
Music, 17–18
Mutuality, 94–99
Mutual vulnerability, 160
My Left Foot (film), 88

N

Neff, K. D., 83
Nelson, Willie, 63
Neutrality, 154. *See also* Multipartiality

O

Objectivity, 42
Observer bias, 43
Oliver, Mary, 44
Orienting empathically to clients, 93–117
  embracing ignorance, 99–102
  eschewing mutuality, 94–99
  not claiming, 114–117
  not judging, 107–114
  not presuming, 103–107
Osler, W., 36, 38, 75
Overgaard, S., 60

P

Paget, Violet (Vernon Lee), 22
Palmer, A. S., 20
Paradigm shift, 52
Parks, Larry, 89–90
Pedersen, P. B., 102
Perry, R., 55, 140
Personal distress, 31–33

Perspective taking, 19, 46, 54, 139
   self-oriented 31, 99
   vs. other-oriented, 31
The Pianist (film), 88
Pitch, in music, 17–18
Pity, 30
Plato, 48
Postempathic stress, 90
Preparation, mindful, 77–81
Prepositions, 21, 23
Preston, S. D., 24–25
Presuming, 103–107
Projecting the imagination, 4, 23, 24, 59, 71, 76, 112, 120, 128, 131, 142, 143, 144, 146
Projecting the self, 21

Q

Questions, asking, 140–145
Quigley, Karen S., 12

R

Reason, and emotion, 48
Receiving, and sending, 82–84. *See also* Tonglen
Redundancy, benefits of, 120–125
Reflection, 126
Refractive interlacing, 148, 150
Reflective listening, 130–131
Refractive listening, 131–137
Reik, T., 4, 65
Relationships
   complementarity of, 66–67
   symmetry of, 66–69
Releasing, 81–82
Resonance, 39, 53, 55–56. *See also* Sympathetic resonance
Resonance fatigue, 37
Ricard, M., 37, 38, 39
Richie, Lionel, 63
Rinpoche, Dzigar Kongtrul, 34
Rituals, 91–92
Rogers, C. R.
   and developing empathic curiosity, 42–43, 54, 65, 69–70
   and orienting empathically to clients, 98, 107, 111–112, 116–117
   and skills of empathic engagement, 119, 124–126, 130, 137, 140, 145
   and therapist self-care, 76

Romeo and Juliet (Shakespeare), 20
Ronaldo, Christiano, 77
Rosenbaum, R., 131
Ross, Diana, 63
Rumi, 84
Russell, J. A., 50n3
Ruthven, K. K., 17

S

Saunders, G., 105, 114
Schindler's List (film), 111
Selective empathy, 113
Self
   circumscribed, 16, 62, 63, 65, 112, 114
   circumscribed sense of, 31, 57, 76
Self and other, 12–17
Self-care. *See* Therapist self-care
Self-compassion, 83
Self identity, body-based, 13
Self-less imagination, 63–66
Self-oriented perspective taking, 99
Self–other boundaries, 56
Sending, 82–84
Serena Williams, 77
Sexual transgressions, 97–99
Shamay-Tsoory, S. G., 47
Shapiro, J., 47
Shared feeling, 30
Sheeran, Ed, 106
Shlien, J., 126
Siegel, D. J., 119
Simile, 61
Simon, Paul, 63
Simulation, 47
Singer, T., 30, 37, 38
Skills of empathic engagement, 119–157
   asking questions and floating hunches, 140–145
   benefits of redundancy, 120–125
   both–and empathizing, 151–157
   challenges in learning, 125–128
   empathic listening, 128–137
   error correction, 137–140
   interlacing, 145–151
Smith, M., 55
Soderbergh, Steven, 137
Sorkin, Aaron, 19, 24
Spending (Gordon), 79
Springsteen, Bruce, 63, 65

Staub, Ervin, 34
Stotland, E., 45
Stress, post-empathic, 90
Strong, Jeremy, 64, 89
Succession (TV series), 89
Suffer, as term, 75
Suzuki, Shunryu (aka Suzuki Roshi), 5, 15, 104, 105
Symmetrical relationships Bateston on, 67–69
Symmetry, of relationships, 66–69
Sympathetic concern, 29–31
Sympathetic resonance, 12, 18, 26–32, 35, 37, 38, 42, 45, 46, 55, 59, 66, 67, 68, 86, 90, 95, 108, 114, 152
    and affective empathy, 45–46
    downregulation of, 74
    and post-empathic stress, 90
    sympathetic concern, vs., 29, 37–38, 55
    as term, 18
Sympathetic resonance, empathy-inflected, 38
Sympathy, 17–21, 25–33, 68, 95
    empathy-inflected, 30, 37, 114

T

Ta, V. P., 54
Taylor, L., 89, 91
Technique, and attitude, 127
Ted Lasso (fictional character), 41
Theory of mind (ToM), 46–47
Therapist self-care, 73–92
    collecting and releasing, 81–82
    including and learning, 84–86
    incorporating imagination-enhanced mindfulness meditation, 86–88
    mindful disengagement, 88–92
    mindful preparation and engagement, 77–81
    receiving and sending, 82–84
This is Us (TV series), 95
Thomas, L., 121
Through the Looking Glass (Carroll), 19–20
Titchener, Edward, 22
ToM (theory of mind), 46–47
Tonglen, 38–39, 82, 84
Townsend, Ed, 106

Trim tabbing, 148
    trim-tab adjustments, 148, 149
    trim-tab refractions, 150, 163
Turner, Tina, 63

U

Uncertainty, 6, 42, 163
University of Massachusetts Medical Center, 77
University of Pennsylvania, 36
Utilization, 91
    and, as utilizing, 46, 87

V

Valence, 50
Vischer, Robert, 21–22
Vulnerability, mutual, 94, 95, 160
    shared vulnerability, 98
    sympathetic vulnerability, 98
    vs. availability, 34, 35, 71, 105, 129, 160

W

Walking in another's shoes, 56–59
Ward, J., 23n2
Warren, J., 85
Warwick, Dionne, 63
"We Are the World" (song), 63
Weil, Simone, 64
Weingarten, Kaethe, 154
"Welcome to the Party" (meditation), 85
Wilkinson, M., 3
Williams, Serena, 91
Wittgenstein, L., 5, 101
Wonder, Stevie, 63
Woods, Tiger, 77
Woolf, Virginia, 25

Y

Yalom, I., 159–160

Z

Zahavi, D., 60
Zaki, J., 53, 74, 88, 152
Zeig, J., 55, 112

About the Author

Douglas Flemons, PhD, LMFT, is professor emeritus of couple and family therapy and former clinical professor of family medicine at Nova Southeastern University. Holding clinical fellow and approved supervisor designations from the American Association for Marriage and Family Therapy, he has taught and supervised clinical graduate students for over 30 years. Dr. Flemons directed a family therapy training clinic for 5 years; he created and—for 6 years—directed his university's student counseling center; and—for 13 years—he codirected the university's Office of Suicide and Violence Prevention.

Dr. Flemons is the author, coauthor, or coeditor of six other books and the author of 60 articles and book chapters, each of which develops and illuminates a systemic approach to learning and practicing brief therapy, clinical hypnosis, suicide assessment, supervision, sex therapy, academic writing, or qualitative research. He is on the editorial board of the *American Journal of Clinical Hypnosis*, which, in 2021, honored him with the Milton H. Erickson Award for Scientific Excellence in Writing on Clinical Hypnosis for his article "Toward a Relational Theory of Hypnosis." He and his wife live in North Carolina.